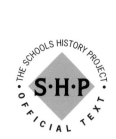

ESSENTIAL

MEDICINE & HEALTH

H TIME

lopment study

/SON

ORE

SON

der Murray

THE HODDER HEADLINE GROUP

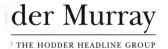
D0183866

The Schools History Project

The project was set up in 1972, with the aim of improving the study of history for students aged 13–16. This involved a reconsideration of the ways in which history contributes to the educational needs of young people. The Project devised new objectives, new criteria for planning and developing courses, and the materials to support them. New examinations requiring new methods of assessment, also had to be developed. These have continued to be popular. The advent of GCSE in 1987 let to the expansion of Project approaches into other syllabuses.

The Schools History Project has been based at Trinity and All Saints College, Leeds, since 1978, from where it supports teachers through a biennial Bulletin, regular INSET, an annual Conference and a website (www.tasc.ac.uk/shp).

Since the National Curriculum was drawn up in 1991, the Project has continued to expand its publications, bringing its ideas to courses for Key Stage 3 as well as a range of GCSE and A level specifications.

Note: The wording and sentence structure of some written sources have been adapted and simplified to make them accessible to all pupils, while faithfully preserving the sense of the original.

Words printed in SMALL CAPITALS are defined in the Glossary on pages 116–117.

© Ian Dawson, Ann Moore, Ian Coulson 2002

First published in 2002
by John Murray (Publishers) Ltd, a member of the Hodder Headline Group
338 Euston Road
London NW1 3BH

Reprinted 2003, 2004, 2005, 2006

Layouts by Liz Rowe
Artwork by Art Construction, Jon Davis/Linden Artists, Janek Matysiak, Chris Rothero/Linden Artists, Steve Smith
Typeset in 13/15 Berthold Walbaum by Wearset Ltd, Boldon, Tyne and Wear
Printed and bound in Great Britain by CPI Bath.

A catalogue entry for this book is available from the British Library.

ISBN-10: 0 7195 8537 6
ISBN-13: 978 0 719 58537 1
Teachers' Resource Book ISBN-10: 0 7195 8538 4
ISBN-13: 978 0 719 58538 8

Acknowledgements

The authors and Publishers would like to thank Lorna Allen for the activity on page 24.

Photo credits
Cover Bridgeman Art Library, London/Royal College of Surgeons, London; **p.2** City of Hereford Archaeological Committee and Mappa Mundi; **p.3** *tr* Mary Evans Picture Library, *bl* British Library (MS Egerton f.53); **p.8** © R. Sheridan/ Ancient Art and Architecture Collection Ltd; **p.13** © The British Museum; **p.15** © The British Museum; **p. 16** © TimePix/ Bust by unidentified artist of Hippocrates (cs. 460–377bc) Greek physician regarded as 'Father of Medicine' from collection of the British Museum; **p.18** © The British Museum; **p.20** © The British Museum; **p.21** © TimePix/ Bust by unidentified artist of Hippocrates (cs. 460–377bc) Greek physician regarded as 'Father of Medicine' from collection of the British Museum; **p.23** *t* Peter Clayton, *b* © Ancient Art and Architecture Collection Ltd, Ronald Sheridan; **p.27** © Ancient Art and Architecture Collection Ltd; **p.29** Wellcome Library, London; **p.37** British Library (MS 42130, f.61r); **p. 44** *l* Ann Ronan Picture Library, *r* Wellcome Library, London; **p. 45** Mary Evans Picture Library; **p. 51** British Library (MS Egerton f.53); **p.55** *t* © Copyright reserved to the Ashmolean Museum, Oxford, *b* Scala, Florence; **p.56** Mary Evans Picture Library; **p.58** Mary Evans Picture Library; **p.60** Reproduced by kind permission of Royal College of Physicians of London; **p.62** Mary Evans Picture Library; **p.63** *l & c* Mary Evans Picture Library, *r* Reproduced by kind permission of Royal College of Physicians of London; **p.65** Wellcome Library, London; **p.66** Mary Evans Picture Library; **p.74** Wellcome Library, London; **p.75** © The British Museum; **p.77** Wellcome Library, London; **p.79** Mary Evans Picture Library; **p.90** Imperial War Museum, London; **p.92** Public Record Office, London (INF 13/140/22); **p.93** Hulton Getty Collection; **p.109** Österreichische Nationalbibliothek, Vienna; **p.110** Wellcome Library, London; **p.111** *t* Hulton Getty Collection, *b* Sean O'Brien, Custom Medical Stock Photo/Science Photo Library.

b = bottom, *c* = centre, *l* = left, *r* = right, *t* = top.

Every effort has been made to trace all copyright holders, but if any have been inadvertently overlooked the Publishers will be pleased to make the necessary arrangements at the first opportunity.

Contents

Introduction

What is a development study?

Skeletons are very useful things. We can learn a lot from them about how people lived in the past. Skeletons can tell us what kinds of food people ate and what illnesses they suffered from. We can even tell how old the people were when they died.

Skeletons like the one on the right tell us that in the past most people died **before they were 40**. Today most of us will live until we are over 70.

So the **big question** in this book is 'Why do we live so much longer nowadays?'

To answer that question you need to look at the topic of medicine and health over a **long period of time**. This kind of historical investigation is called a *development study*. This development study investigates medicine and health since the time of the ancient Egyptians, 5000 years ago. It investigates:

1 **CONTINUITIES** – the things that stayed the same for many years
2 **CHANGES** – the great ideas and discoveries that changed medicine and health
3 **REASONS** – why medicine and health stayed the same or changed.

Once you have studied these things you will be able to answer our **big question**:

> Why do we live so much longer nowadays?

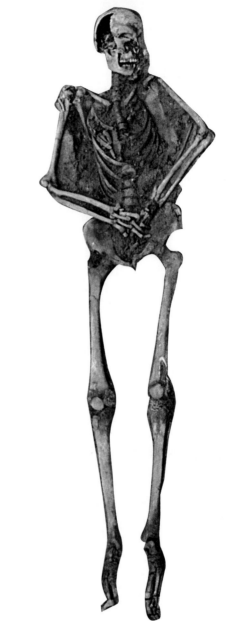

▲ **SOURCE 1** The skeleton of a victim of the Black Death, a disease that killed nearly half the people of Britain in the 1300s

■ ACTIVITY

Here are the main reasons why medicine and health have changed. Work in pairs and choose one of the reasons. Think of why it might have helped to change medicine and health.

■ Attitudes and religious beliefs
■ War
■ Governments
■ Communications
■ Science and technology
■ Individual genius

Your pathway

Chapter 1 Medicine in Egypt, Greece and Rome

Find out
- about the first doctors
- some good ideas about causes of disease
- why the Romans went to the baths.

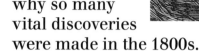
A healthy army means a healthy empire!

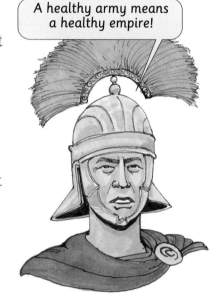

Chapter 2 Medicine in the Middle Ages 400–1350

Find out why the Black Death killed half the people in Europe.

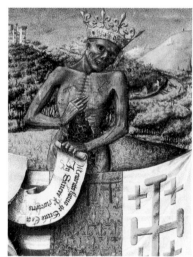

Chapter 3 Renaissance Medicine 1350–1750

Find out about three really important medical discoveries – and why people were still no healthier!

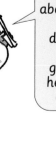

Read all about it! Great medical discoveries! Nobody getting any healthier for centuries!

Chapter 4 Medicine during the Industrial Revolution 1750–1900

- Choose the four greatest Medical Marvels for the Hall of Fame!
- Think about why so many vital discoveries were made in the 1800s.

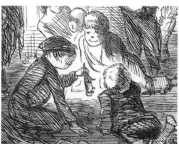

Chapter 5 Medicine since 1900

NHS, DNA – what do these initials mean and why are they so important to every one of us?

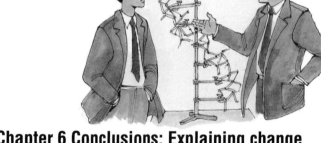

Chapter 6 Conclusions: Explaining change and continuity in medicine and health

The answers come together! Now you can explain why we live so much longer nowadays.

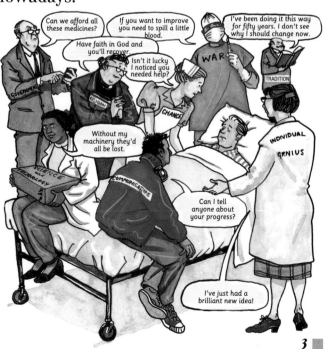

The starting point: prehistoric times

The villagers in the picture opposite lived 7000 years ago.
They were lucky if they lived to be 40. Can you work out
why they died so young?

■ ACTIVITY

1 Copy the table below. Use the information around the picture on
page 5 to fill in the table.

	What was the illness/ medical problem?	How was the illness treated?	Did the treatment work?
Girl			
Woman			
Boy			
Man			

2 Use the information in your table to answer the questions in the
diagram below.
3 Use your answers to questions 1 and 2 to explain why you think
people died so young 7000 years ago.
4 How would each of these illnesses be treated today?

Who treated the sick?

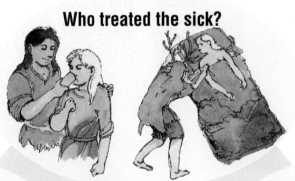

How did they treat the sick?

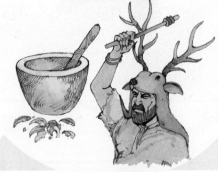

Medicine in prehistoric times

What did they think caused disease?

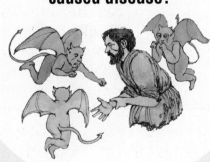

1 The **girl** has a sore throat. This is a common illness and her mother has a good REMEDY that she learned from her own mother. She gives the girl a drink made from herbs and honey and the girl soon feels better.

2 The **woman** is pregnant. She feels sick and tired all the time. She has a sharp pain in her side. The medicine man puts CHARMS on her forehead and says prayers to the gods but she is not getting better. When her baby is born in three weeks' time she will die from bleeding, and the baby will die too.

4 The **man** has cut his hand on the flint knife and it is red and painful. He has smeared the cut with healing herbs but he thinks that an evil spirit has got into his body through the cut. In ten days' time his jaws will lock together. The medicine man will drill a hole in his skull to release the evil spirit but it won't work and the man will die.

3 The **boy** broke his ankle last year. His father covered it in mud and leaves until the mud set hard. The break healed but the boy still walks with a limp.

This chapter investigates medicine and health in three great empires, Egypt, Greece and Rome. Each of these empires had a BIG MEDICAL IDEA. Here they are:

Egypt – specialist doctors learned from experience

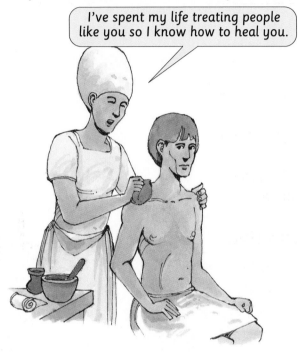

I've spent my life treating people like you so I know how to heal you.

Rome – PUBLIC HEALTH: stopping the spread of disease

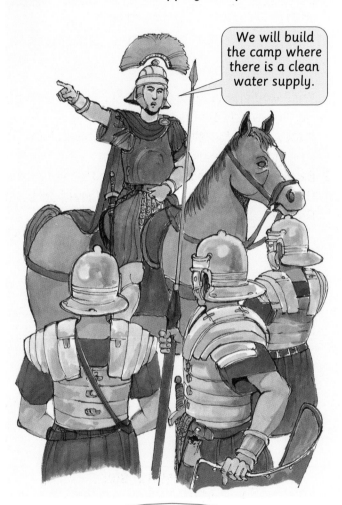

We will build the camp where there is a clean water supply.

Greece – the four HUMOURS: a logical reason for illness

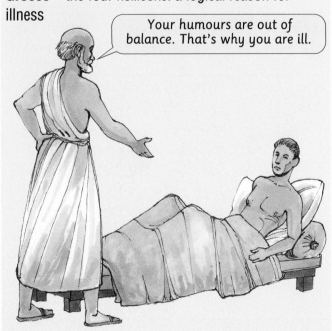

Your humours are out of balance. That's why you are ill.

Why were these three BIG IDEAS so important if people still didn't live longer?

Timeline of the great empires

BRITAIN			Stonehenge						AD43 Roman conquest of Britain	
	THE EGYPTIAN EMPIRE									
							THE GREEK EMPIRE			
								THE ROMAN EMPIRE		

3000BC   2000BC   1000BC   0   AD500

■ DISCUSS

1 What evidence is there on page 6 that people in Egypt, Greece and Rome tried to help the sick?

2 If they did try to help the sick, why do you think people did not live as long as we do today?

3 Below is how you could have completed your diagram from page 4. Do you think the situation will be different for Egypt, Greece and Rome?

Who treated the sick?

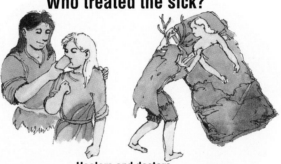

Healers and doctors
Most illnesses were treated by mothers and other women. Medicine men tried to cure more difficult illnesses that the women could not cure.

How did they treat the sick?

Medicine in prehistoric times

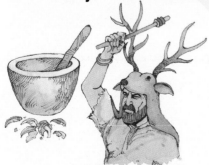

Treatments
Herbs and other remedies were used for some problems. Magic charms and spells were used for others.

What did they think caused disease?

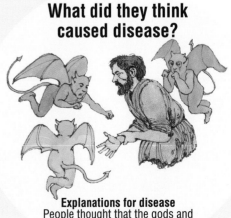

Explanations for disease
People thought that the gods and evil spirits caused diseases.

1.1 Egypt *Doctors – the Egyptians' big idea!*

The Egyptians' big idea was specialist doctors. Over the next four pages you are going to find out more about these doctors and the treatments they used. You will decide how to cure the PHARAOH of his illnesses.

Who treated the sick in Ancient Egypt?

The Egyptians had specialist doctors who were also priests.

▼ **SOURCE 1** Tomb painting of Irj, priest PHYSICIAN to the pharaoh. He was a 'Palace doctor, Superintendent of the court physicians, Palace eye physician, Palace physician of the belly, One understanding internal fluids, Guardian of the anus'

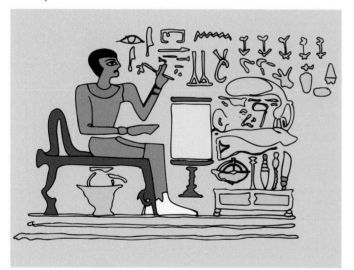

▼ **SOURCE 2** Sekhmet, goddess of war. Egyptians believed that she caused and cured EPIDEMICS

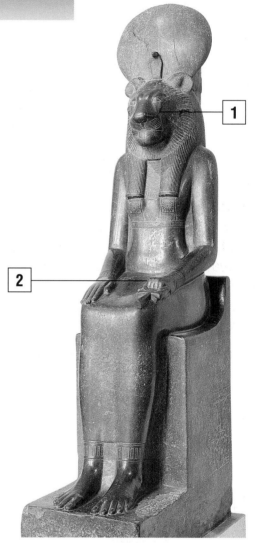

Find…

1 Look at Source 2. It contains numbered symbols. Match the symbols to these explanations.

■ A lion's head. This shows Sekhmet's anger. She is bringing PLAGUE upon the people.

■ An ankh ☥ . This is a holy symbol of life. It shows that Sekhmet forgives people and brings life again!

What did the Egyptians think caused diseases?

These doctors did not know about GERMS so they had to think of other reasons why people became ill. Sometimes they thought it was the fault of angry gods like Sekhmet. But they had other ideas too.

Blocked channels

The Egyptians knew about the heart, liver, lungs and brain because they removed them when they EMBALMED people who had died. That was when they noticed that the blood flowed through channels (we call them veins and arteries) from the heart to every part of the body. They thought that these channels also carried life-giving air. They decided that people became ill when the channels in their bodies became blocked. For example, undigested food rotting in the bowels would cause blockages in the channels and this made people ill.

▼ **SOURCE 3** Egyptian ideas about how blocked channels cause disease

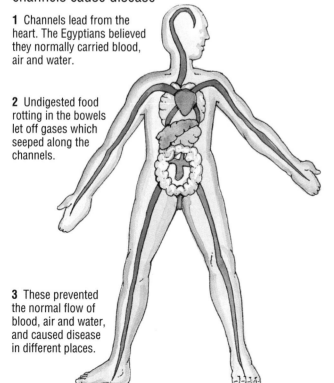

1 Channels lead from the heart. The Egyptians believed they normally carried blood, air and water.

2 Undigested food rotting in the bowels let off gases which seeped along the channels.

3 These prevented the normal flow of blood, air and water, and caused disease in different places.

▼ **SOURCE 4** As soon as someone died, his or her brain, liver and other organs were taken out. Then the body was embalmed or mummified. You can find out why they did this on page 13. Embalming helped the Egyptians to find out a lot about the body

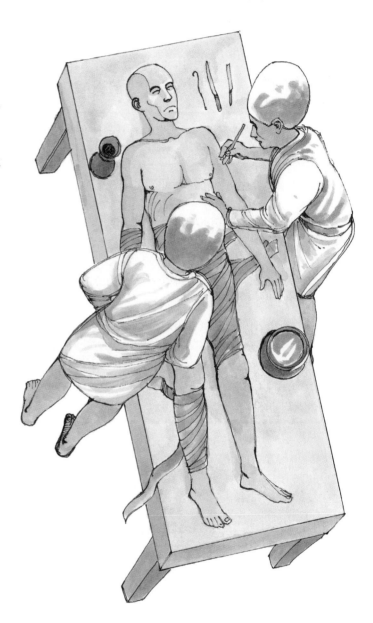

■ **DISCUSS**

2 How did the Egyptians learn about parts of the body?

3 The Egyptians explained illness in two ways. What were they?

How did the Egyptians treat illnesses?

In Source 1 on page 8 you can see some of the tools used by Irj. You can tell he must have done some surgery. There were two kinds of doctor who used different remedies:

- priest physicians who used common sense and herbal remedies
- priest magicians who used supernatural remedies, such as prayers, charms and spells.

■ ACTIVITY

Treating the pharaoh

1 Work with a partner for this activity. One of you is a priest physician, the other is a priest magician. You have to treat the pharaoh. He is old and has several illnesses:

- a broken nose
- a sore eye
- stomach ache.

   Work together to prepare a presentation, explaining how you will treat each illness. The pharoah will expect you to use a combination of natural and supernatural remedies. He believes in both. Use the information in Sources 5–7 to help you. You can use drawings, text, video or tape.

▼ **SOURCE 5** From the Edwin Smith Papyrus, a collection of Egyptian medical documents written about 1600BC. The PAPYRUS lists 48 cases of SURGERY, each with a careful description of DIAGNOSIS and treatment

Instructions for treating a broken nose
Diagnosis
If you examine a man whose nose is part squashed in, part swollen and both his nostrils are bleeding then you should say, 'You have a broken nose and this is an ailment [health problem] which I can treat.'

Treatment
You should clean his nose with two plugs of linen and then insert two plugs soaked in grease into his nostrils. You should make him rest until the swelling has gone down, you should bandage his nose with stiff rolls of linen and treat him with lint every day until he recovers.

▼ **SOURCE 6** Two treatments described in Egyptian medical documents written between 1900 and 1500BC

Treatment 1: For any disease
This charm will protect you against evil spirits. It is made from evil-smelling herbs and garlic and from honey which is sweet for people but horrible for spirits, from a fishtail and a rag and a backbone of a perch.

Treatment 2: For a diseased eye
To clear up the pus:
honey, balm from Mecca and gum ammoniac.
To treat its discharge:
frankincense, myrrh, yellow ochre.
To treat the growth:
red ochre, malachite, honey.

▼ **SOURCE 7** The Greek historian Herodotus, 450BC

For all diseases
For three successive days every month, the Egyptians PURGE themselves [take potions which make them sick or have diarrhoea] ... for they think that all diseases come from the foods they eat.

Did these treatments work?

This cartoon is based on information in *The Medical Skills of Ancient Egypt* by J. Worth Estes, published in 1989

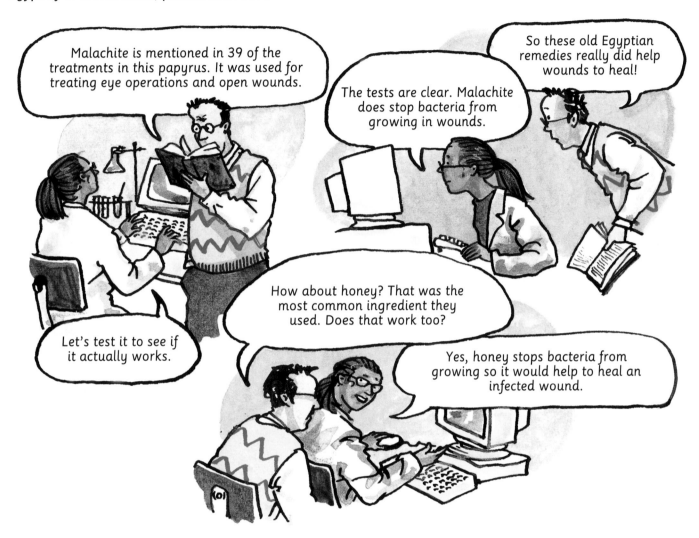

■ DISCUSS

2 Which two treatments are the scientists investigating?

3 Why did these treatments work?

4 The Egyptians did not know how these treatments worked (because they did not know about BACTERIA), so why did they carry on using them?

5 Look back at your treatment of the pharaoh in the activity on page 10. Is there anything that you would now like to change?

1.2 Egypt

How did the Egyptians' way of life help them to develop medical ideas?

> To understand Egyptian medicine it helps to know more about what Egypt was like. Over the next four pages you will look closely at Egyptian life and complete your own table explaining the changes in Egyptian medicine.

Egypt is a country in North Africa. Five thousand years ago Egypt had one of the greatest civilisations in the world.

Here is a summary of key points you have learned so far about Egyptian doctors and medicine.

The Egyptians had doctors who were also priests.

They knew about many parts of the body's ANATOMY, such as the heart, lungs, liver and brain.

Egyptian doctors and medicine

They believed illness was caused by the gods or when the channels in the body became blocked.

They treated illnesses with herbal remedies, prayer and magic charms, simple surgery or by purging the body.

■ ACTIVITY 1

Why did Egyptian medicine develop as it did? Copy this table and fill in the second column as you read about Egyptian life on pages 13–15.

The Egyptian way of life	How this helped to change medicine
1 Pharaohs were wealthy and powerful.	
2 The Egyptians developed writing.	
3 Their religion said that priests had to be clean at all times.	
4 The bodies of the dead were opened up for embalming for the after-life.	
5 The Egyptian farmers irrigated their fields using water channels.	
6 The Egyptians traded with other countries.	

Pharaohs

Egypt was ruled by pharaohs. They were worshipped as kings and also as gods. Egyptians had many gods, but the pharaoh was always the most important god.

The pharaohs were also fabulously wealthy. They lived in wonderful palaces. When the pharaohs died they were buried in huge tombs and pyramids. The stories of their lives were painted on the walls of their tombs, or written on papyrus scrolls. Historians have found out a great deal about Egyptian medicine from tomb paintings such as Source 1 on page 8.

Priests

Pharaohs were advised by priests. Priests could read and write. Their religion said that priests had to stay clean all the time. They washed themselves every day, shaved their bodies and drank from clean bronze cups. Sometimes the priests were also doctors. The pharaohs encouraged these priest doctors to develop their skills.

Because the pharaohs trusted the priest doctors and paid their wages, other wealthy Egyptians trusted them, too. They copied the priests' habits of cleanliness and tried many of their remedies and treatments.

The priests wrote down *all* of their remedies so that other people could copy and learn from them.

Embalming

The Egyptians believed that people had a life after death and would need their bodies in the after-life. As soon as someone died, his or her body was cut open. The brain and other organs were taken out. Then the body was sewn up again and embalmed (mummified). They had to do this very quickly, before the body began to rot in the hot Egyptian climate. Embalming helped the Egyptians to find out a great deal about the body and its organs. As they tried to find the best methods of preserving a body, they learned more about spices, ointments and surgery.

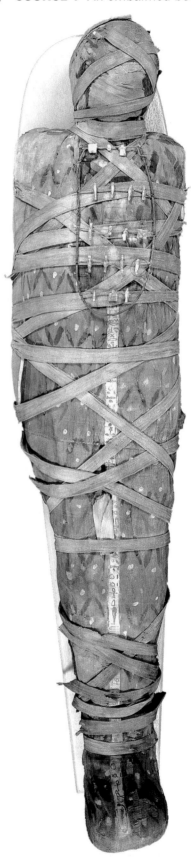

▼ **SOURCE 1** An embalmed body

■ **ACTIVITY 2**

Now fill in rows 1–4 of your table.

The River Nile and farming

The longest river in Africa, the River Nile, flowed through Egypt. Egyptian farmers depended on the River Nile. They were very successful farmers. They dug channels from the Nile to carry water to their fields. Even during the hot summer months they could still water their crops. However, the channels sometimes got blocked. Then the crops died because they had no water.

The Egyptians noticed what happened to their crops and they thought that the body must work like this. The human heart was like the Nile and the rest of the body like the crops. Therefore the body must have channels carrying blood from the heart to the rest of the body. If the channels became blocked then people became sick.

▼ **SOURCE 2** A wall painting from the tomb of Nakht, a priest and royal official. It shows him supervising work on the temple lands

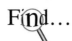 **Find...**

1 Find . . . in Source 2:

- people sowing seeds and ploughing the land
- people harvesting crops into huge baskets
- people threshing corn
- people gathering seeds into small containers
- Nakht pouring seeds on to a table loaded with fruit, vegetables, birds, legs of beef
- butchers cutting up a dead cow.

■ **DISCUSS**

2 Who do you think the food piled up on the table in Source 2 was for?
3 How does this source show that farming and the Nile were very important to the Egyptians?
4 In your opinion, was the Egyptian explanation for the causes of disease sensible? Give at least two reasons to support your opinion.
5 Now fill in row 5 of your table.

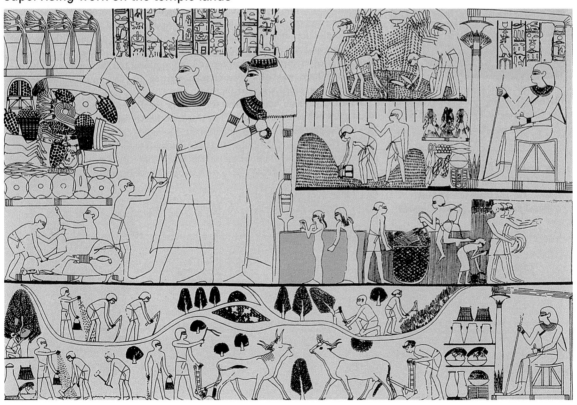

Trade with other countries

Because the Egyptians had such a good lifestyle and no worries about food, they were able to develop new skills. People made tools, instruments, jewellery and furniture. They learned to sail and build ships to travel along the Nile. This led to trade with India, China and other countries. The Egyptians exchanged their goods for herbs, plants and ointments that were known to have healing properties. Priest doctors used them to cure people.

▼ **SOURCE 3** Traders from Syria paying their respects to the pharaoh, *c.* 1400BC. (The pharaoh can not be seen on this preserved part of the painting.)

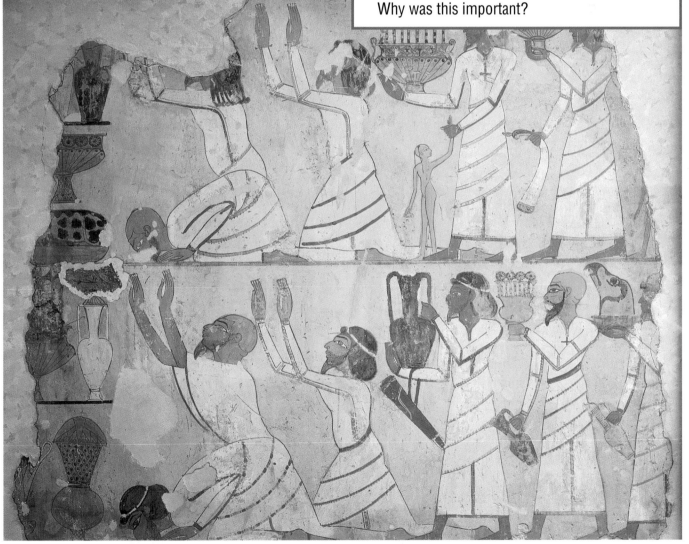

Find…

6 Find . . . in Source 3:

■ small jars holding precious oils
■ large jars holding wine
■ evidence that the pharaoh was powerful.

■ **ACTIVITY**

7 Fill in row 6 of your table.
8 On page 2 you saw six reasons why medicine has changed. Which reason was most important in changing medicine in ancient Egypt? Give two reasons for your choice.
9 The Egyptians' big idea was specialist doctors. Why was this important?

1.3 Greece

The theory of the four humours – the Greeks' big idea!

The Egyptians and the Greeks knew each other well. They traded with each other across the Mediterranean Sea and the Greeks borrowed many medical ideas from the Egyptians. However, the Greeks also had lots of new ideas. The most important was the idea or theory of the four humours. This theory affected how doctors treated sick people all over Europe for the next 2000 years! In this section you will write a speech explaining this very important idea.

What was Hippocrates' big idea?

1 My name is Hippocrates. My BIG IDEA explains why people become ill. It's because their humours, the liquids in their body, are out of balance.

2 There are four humours in the body. I have watched people carefully when they are ill. One of the four humours often comes out of the body, as you see below.

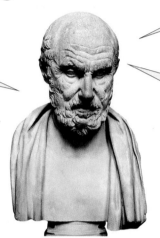

3 I think that people stay healthy when they have just the right amount of each humour in their bodies. But if the humours become unbalanced and people have too much or too little of one of them, that's when they become ill.

4 My discovery is important because it shows that some illnesses have natural causes. I disagree with people who say that all illnesses are caused by the gods. If so, how can we do anything to help the patients? Only the gods can make them better! But if an illness has a natural cause we can find a way to make the patient better – that is why my discovery is so important.

Blood
People sometimes cough up blood or have nosebleeds.

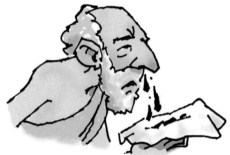

Phlegm
People often sneeze or cough up slimy, revolting phlegm.

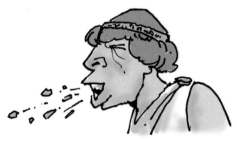

Yellow bile
People often vomit up their half-digested food after a meal.

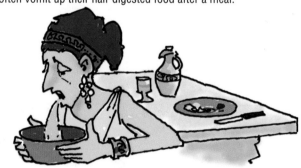

Black bile
People sometimes vomit even when they have not eaten. This vomit is a dark, evil-smelling liquid.

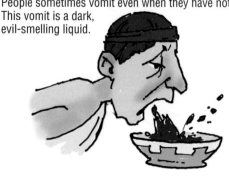

The four seasons

Hippocrates linked these four humours to the four seasons. Here, again, he was using careful observations. Although his conclusions were wrong he was at least looking for natural explanations.

▼ **SOURCE 1** How Greek doctors could link the seasons and the humours

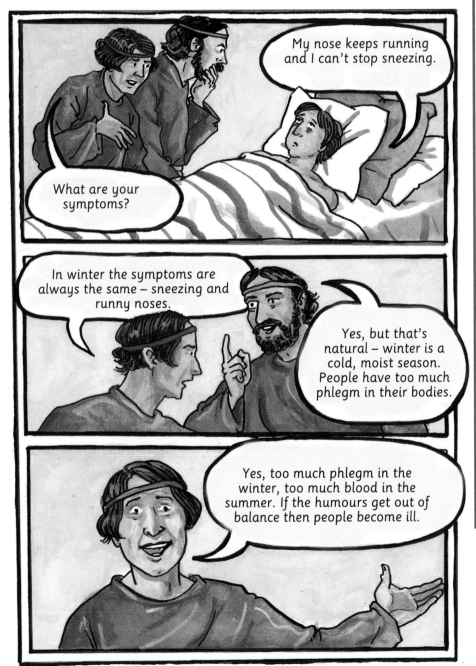

How did the Greeks treat illnesses?

Hippocrates' new idea became very popular. People could see the logic of it and work it out for themselves. Hippocrates encouraged doctors to use his ideas as the basis for treatments. Many of the treatments worked because they were logical. Pages 18–21 help you to investigate these treatments and you can use them to write the second half of your speech.

Careful observation

Hippocrates said that since the gods did not cause all diseases, doctors could work out how to cure people. Greek doctors began to OBSERVE their patients very carefully. This helped them to diagnose what was wrong with them. They wrote down what they saw and worked out which humours were unbalanced and what treatments were needed.

▼ **SOURCE 2** The tomb of a Greek doctor, shown examining a child

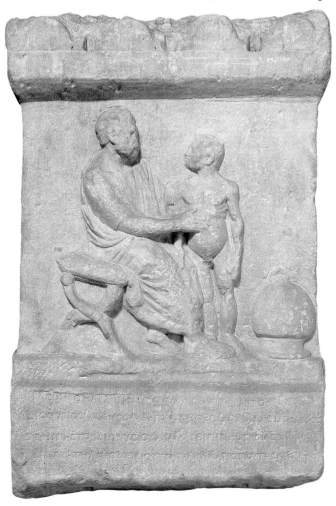

■ **ACTIVITY**

1 Draw up a chart with two columns, one headed 'Natural diagnoses or treatments' and the other headed 'Supernatural diagnoses or treatments'. As you work through this next section, list each remedy or treatment that is mentioned under the correct heading.

■ **DISCUSS**

2 What can you learn from Source 2 about:
   a) Greek doctors and their methods?
   b) Greek attitudes to doctors?

Rest, exercise and pray!

Greek doctors usually advised their patients that the best way to get well was to restore the balance of the four humours in their body. This meant *resting* or *changing their diet*. As they got better patients were advised to take *regular exercise*. All patients were told to *keep clean*. Doctors had observed their patients and had worked out that all these things seemed to help their patients to get better.

At Greek temples there were also baths and gymnasiums. They were a good example of how the Greeks combined natural and supernatural treatments. People prayed to the gods (supernatural treatment). At the same time they rested, bathed and exercised (natural treatments).

▼ **SOURCE 3** Advice from the Greek doctor Diocles, 390BC

After arising he should rub the whole body with oil. Then he should wash face and eyes using pure water.

Long walks before meals clear out the body, prepare it for receiving food and give it more power for digesting.

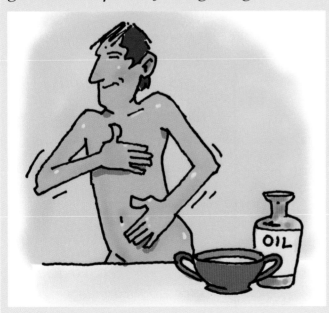

▼ **SOURCE 4** From *A Programme for Health*, one of the books in the Hippocratic Collection of medical books, 400–200BC

In winter, people should eat as much as possible and drink as little as possible – unwatered wine, bread, roast meat and few vegetables. This will keep the body hot and dry. In summer they should drink more and eat less – watered wine, barley cakes and boiled meat so that the body will stay cold and moist. Walking should be fast in winter and slow in summer.

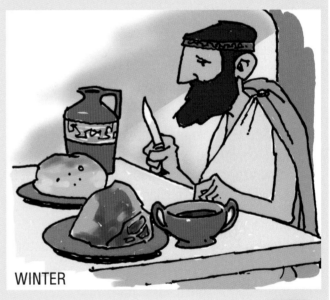

WINTER

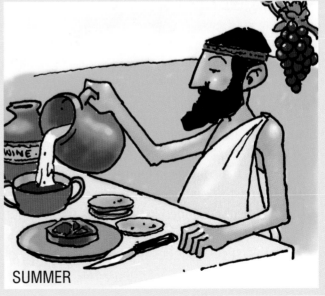

SUMMER

Vomiting and purging

If patients were still ill, they could be prescribed more treatments to restore their unbalanced humours. They could be made to vomit or to purge (empty) their bowels or else doctors could BLEED them. A cut was made in the patient's arm and blood was caught in a small bowl or cup.

▼ **SOURCE 5** A bleeding cup

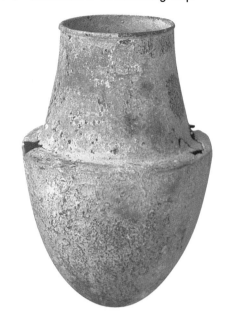

■ ACTIVITY 1

Each of the sources you have seen is important evidence about Greek medicine. Use this activity to make revision notes.

1 Here is a list of five different ways in which Greek doctors observed their patients:

- inspecting urine
- inspecting faeces
- feeling temperature
- listening to breathing
- asking the patient questions.

Copy Source 6 into the centre of a page in your exercise book. Use the list to help you to label each day with the method of observation the doctor must have used to get the information (two have been done for you).

2 Examine Source 2 on page 18. What three methods of observation do you think the doctor is using?

3 Examine Source 3 on page 19. Is Diocles advising natural or supernatural treatments? Explain your answer carefully.

4 Read Source 4 on page 19. Explain how this advice will keep the humours balanced and the patient healthy.

1 he must have asked the patient questions

2 he must have inspected urine

■ ACTIVITY 2

5 ■ Divide into two teams for this activity.
■ Each team takes it in turn to choose one of Sources 7–10, or one of the sources in the rest of the section.
■ One person in the team (or more if necessary) acts out the treatment described in the source for the opposite team.
■ The opposition have to guess which source it is.
■ For each correct guess win 5 points. For each incorrect guess lose 5 points.

▼ **SOURCE 6** A patient's case history from the Hippocratic Collection, 400–200BC

Silenius began with pains in his belly, heavy head and stiff neck.

First day: *he vomited, his urine was black, he was thirsty, his tongue dry and he did not sleep.*

Second day: *slightly* DELIRIOUS.

Sixth day: *slight perspiration; head and feet cold, no discharge from the bowels, no urine.*

Eighth day: *cold sweat all over; red rashes; severe diarrhoea.*

Eleventh day: *Breathing slow and heavy. He died. He was aged about twenty.*

Now you know all about my big idea – the theory of the four humours.

It was important because instead of blaming illness on the gods it was a natural explanation for illness. If there is a natural cause the doctors can really help their patients with natural treatments, instead of just praying to the gods.

People carried on believing in my idea for thousands of years – as you will see!

▼ **SOURCE 7** From the Greek doctor Diocles, 390BC

He should rub his teeth inside and outside with the fingers using fine peppermint powder and cleaning the teeth of remnants of food.

▼ **SOURCE 8** From the Greek doctor Diocles, 390BC

He should anoint nose and ears inside, preferably with well-perfumed oil.

▼ **SOURCE 9** From the Hippocratic Collection, 400–200BC

If the pain is under the DIAPHRAGM, clear the bowels, with a medicine made from black hellebore, cumin or other fragrant herbs.

■ ACTIVITY 3

6 Now it's time to finish the speech you began on page 17. You need to tell the doctors about the treatments that are best. You could include some of these points in your speech:

■ why observation is important
■ why patients need to rest and exercise carefully
■ why the sick often need to change their diet in order to get better
■ why purging and vomiting help people to get better
■ how your treatments are based on your theory of the four humours.

■ DISCUSS

7 Hippocrates was wrong about the causes of illness. He did not know about germs or VIRUSES. So why do you think his idea was so important if he was wrong?

▼ **SOURCE 10** From the Hippocratic Collection, 400–200BC

A bath will help PNEUMONIA as it soothes pain and brings up phlegm.

1.4 Greece *A visit to an Asclepion*

Don't think that all the Greeks thought like Hippocrates. At the same time as Hippocrates was developing his ideas, other Greeks still believed that the gods caused and cured illnesses. They believed in Asclepius, the God of Healing. On these two pages you can find out what happened at an Asclepion.

The main Greek gods of healing were Asclepius and his daughters, Panacea and Hygeia. Temples were built, dedicated to Asclepius and his daughters. People went there to rest, exercise, eat a healthy diet (natural treatment) and be cured magically (supernatural treatment) by Asclepius. The Greeks believed that when they went to sleep, the gods would visit them. Source 1 tells you what they thought would happen; Source 2 is a carved stone panel of Asclepius, as the Greeks imagined him.

▼ **SOURCE 1** A visit to an Asclepion. The story comes from a play by the Greek writer Aristophanes, around 400BC. Aristophanes put a lot of realistic description into his plays

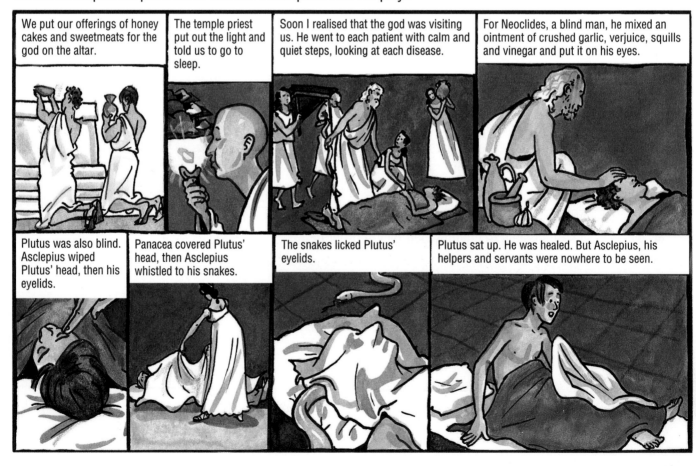

We put our offerings of honey cakes and sweetmeats for the god on the altar.

The temple priest put out the light and told us to go to sleep.

Soon I realised that the god was visiting us. He went to each patient with calm and quiet steps, looking at each disease.

For Neoclides, a blind man, he mixed an ointment of crushed garlic, verjuice, squills and vinegar and put it on his eyes.

Plutus was also blind. Asclepius wiped Plutus' head, then his eyelids.

Panacea covered Plutus' head, then Asclepius whistled to his snakes.

The snakes licked Plutus' eyelids.

Plutus sat up. He was healed. But Asclepius, his helpers and servants were nowhere to be seen.

We know from written evidence that many people who visited the temples did get better. This was probably because they were resting, exercising properly and eating healthily. These were the natural treatments that the Greeks received.

Another reason why many Greeks recovered from their illnesses might be that they really *believed* that they would get better.

▼ **SOURCE 3** A votive or 'thank you' stone. This one was put up by a visitor to the Asclepion to give thanks to the gods for being cured of a problem with the leg or foot

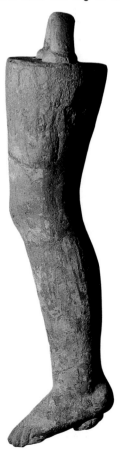

▼ **SOURCE 2** Asclepius healing the sick

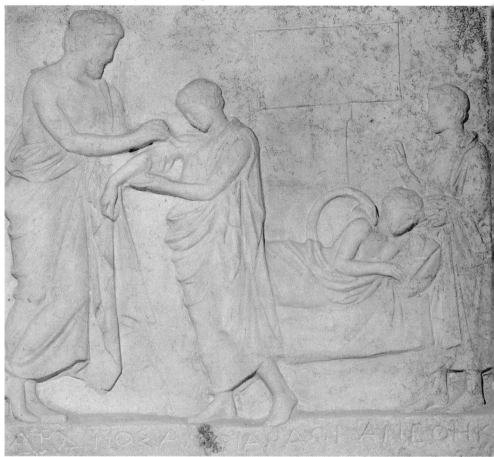

■ **ACTIVITY**

Imagine you have returned from the Temple of Asclepius. You went there sure that you were about to die, because your constant headaches were so bad. Miraculously you have been cured.

1 Design a votive stone that will go up in the garden of the temple.
2 Write your thanks to Asclepius on this votive stone. Explain your illness and describe how it has been cured.

Find...

3 Find ... in Source 2:

■ the snake, 'licking' a patient better
■ Asclepius putting ointment on the boy's arm
■ Panacea watching over the sick man.

1.5 ROME *Public health – the Romans' big idea!*

Your third empire! The Roman empire. The Romans' big idea was public health! They spent a lot of time and money providing clean water and public baths for the people who lived in Roman towns. On the next four pages you can see exactly what they did and why they did it. At the end you will see if you know enough to get the job advertised below.

■ ACTIVITY 1

You are applying for the job of a Public Health Inspector in a Roman town. Complete the questionnaire below using the information on pages 25–27 and explain the reason for each choice. The person who gives the most correct answers and the best explanations will get the job.

OFFICIAL QUESTIONNAIRE

FOR THE POST OF STAFF INSPECTOR, REPORTING TO CORPULENTUS GROSSUS: SENIOR PUBLIC HEALTH ADMINISTRATOR, PLUMBRIAN REGION

1 **You have been instructed to build a new Roman settlement. Do you**
   a) choose a site with plenty of fresh air and spring water
   b) choose an old settlement near marshy land – this will be much quicker and easier.

2 **Your town is growing bigger – you don't have enough water. Do you**
   a) pray for rain
   b) limit the townspeople to one bucket a day and insist that they pay for it
   c) build channels to bring fresh water into the town.

3 **Your town has been given money for new buildings. Do you**
   a) decide to build public baths, lavatories and sewers to protect the health of your citizens
   b) build a theatre to entertain local people because they need to relax after a hard day's work.

4 **Roman soldiers have been injured near your town. Do you**
   a) build a new hospital for wounded soldiers
   b) stop trying to defend the empire
   c) improve the training of your soldiers because they don't know how to defend themselves.

5 **You have built new baths in the town. Will you**
   a) make a very low entry charge so everyone can keep clean
   b) have a high entry charge so that only the wealthy can use the baths.

6 **You have many poor people and slaves in your town who sometimes fall ill. Do you**
   a) ignore them because they are an unimportant section of your population
   b) pay for a doctor to treat them
   c) tell them to pray to the gods more often.

How did the Romans keep their army healthy?

The Roman empire was much bigger than the Egyptian or Greek empires. It reached from Italy into Germany, Spain and Britain and across to North Africa. The Romans built up their huge empire thanks to their very powerful and disciplined army. The Romans worked hard to improve public health because they had to keep the army healthy to defend the empire.

As the Roman army travelled across Europe and North Africa, its leaders noticed that every time the soldiers camped near to swamps and marshes they became ill with MALARIA. Although they did not know about germs, the Romans realised that there was a connection between dirty water and disease. So they built their forts and camps well away from marshes and swamps. They tried to build near fresh water. If that was not possible, their engineers designed AQUEDUCTS to bring fresh water from the rivers to the camps. Each fort had a bath house with drains and fresh water.

The Romans also built hospitals for their soldiers. This meant that the soldiers got the best treatments possible from trained SURGEONS and doctors. These treatments were very similar to those used by the Greeks. They mostly depended on herbal medicine, simple surgery, or rest, diet and exercise. Of course the soldiers, like everybody else, also used magic charms or prayed to the gods to be cured.

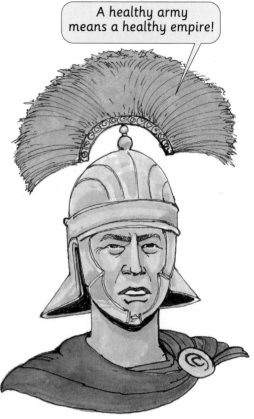

A healthy army means a healthy empire!

▼ **SOURCE 2** One Roman soldier wrote:

Soldiers must not remain for too long near unhealthy marshes. A soldier . . . must not drink swamp water.

▼ **SOURCE 1** A plan of a Roman army hospital built in Scotland. There was room for 240 patients and there was also an operating theatre, kitchens and baths

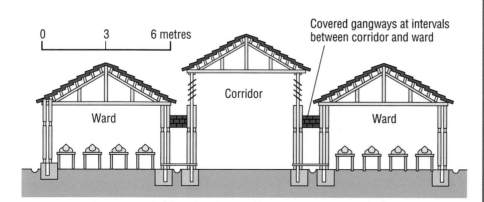

0 3 6 metres

Covered gangways at intervals between corridor and ward

Ward

Corridor

Ward

■ ACTIVITY 2

The Romans wanted to keep their soldiers healthy and fighting-fit. If they did not have a fit army they would lose their empire. Using the information on this page, make a list of all the methods they used to keep their soldiers healthy.

25 ■

How did the Romans keep their towns healthy?

These practical methods and ideas helped the Roman army to stay fit and healthy. People soon realised that they could use the same ideas in their homes in Roman cities or when they were building new towns or villas. As soon as the Romans realised how important it was to have fresh water, baths, hospitals and sewers to keep people healthy, they made sure that *all* their new towns followed the same pattern.

> We have lots of slaves to do the building but it still takes a lot of money and careful organisation.

> It's not just the army that need to be healthy! We Romans are the first government to care about improving the people's health.

▼ **SOURCE 3** How the Romans improved public health

A Roman engineer always . . .

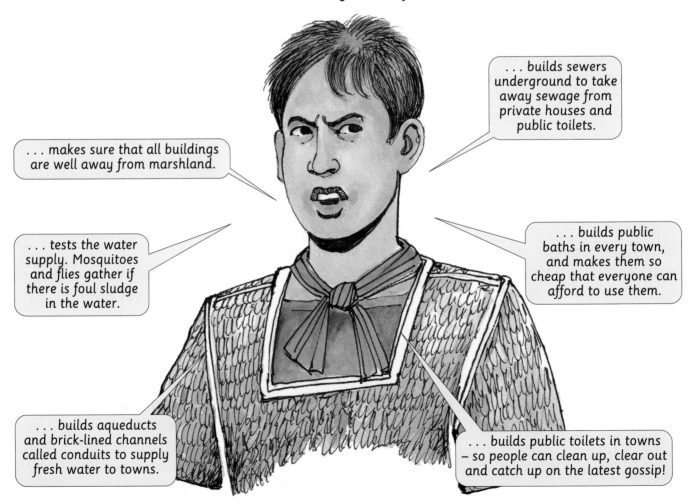

> . . . makes sure that all buildings are well away from marshland.

> . . . builds sewers underground to take away sewage from private houses and public toilets.

> . . . tests the water supply. Mosquitoes and flies gather if there is foul sludge in the water.

> . . . builds public baths in every town, and makes them so cheap that everyone can afford to use them.

> . . . builds aqueducts and brick-lined channels called conduits to supply fresh water to towns.

> . . . builds public toilets in towns – so people can clean up, clear out and catch up on the latest gossip!

▼ **SOURCE 4** A Roman aqueduct and how it worked

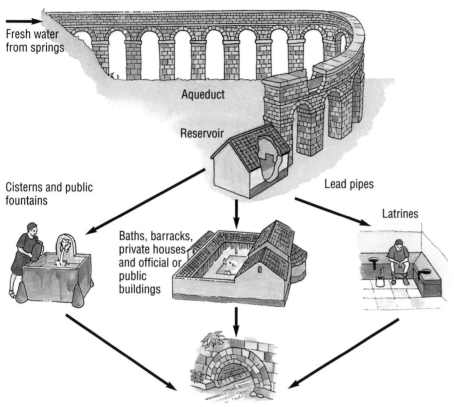

Fresh water from springs

Aqueduct

Reservoir

Cisterns and public fountains

Lead pipes

Baths, barracks, private houses and official or public buildings

Latrines

Sewers emptying into river

▼ **SOURCE 6** A Roman author, Marcus Varro

When building a house or farm, especial care should be taken to place it at the foot of a wooded hill where it is exposed to health-giving winds. Care should be taken when there are swamps in the neighbourhood because certain tiny creatures which cannot be seen by the eyes breed there. These float through the air and enter the body through the mouth and nose and cause serious diseases.

▼ **SOURCE 5** The Roman baths at Bath in Somerset. The baths have been preserved and you can visit them today to walk where the Romans walked

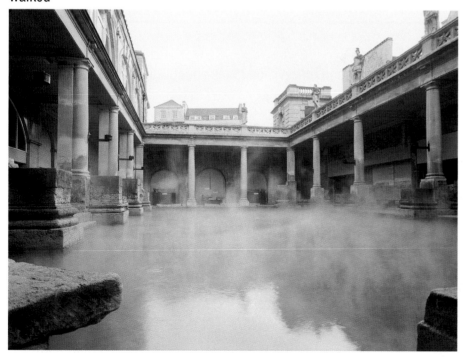

■ **DISCUSS**

Study Source 6.

1 What do you think the tiny creatures would be called nowadays?
2 Do you think the Roman reasoning was sensible?

1.6 Rome — *Why was Galen so important?*

Galen was a famous doctor in Rome. These two pages help you to decide why he was so important and also help you to build up a diagram to use for revision because you will certainly need to know about him for your exam.

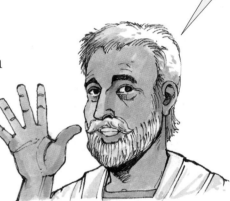

> I am more important than all the public health inspectors and engineers in Rome! I am the most important person in the history of medicine – so pay attention to these pages!

Galen's ideas

Galen was born in AD129 in Greece. He began studying medicine when he was sixteen. He spent a long time as a surgeon at a GLADIATORS' school. The gladiators often suffered stab wounds and broken bones. Galen learned a lot about anatomy and treatments.

When he was 33 Galen travelled to Rome. He soon became the Emperor's doctor. He followed Hippocrates' ideas but also had new ideas of his own.

Old ideas

> I believe in Hippocrates' methods.
> - Most diseases are caused when the humours are out of balance.
> - We must observe our patients carefully and record their symptoms before deciding how to treat them.

New idea 1: the treatment of opposites

> But I have a new idea that builds on the theory of the four humours. We must use opposites to balance up the humours and treat illness. For example, if a man has a cold and is sneezing and coughing up phlegm we must treat him with the opposite to cold phlegm. Give him hot fiery pepper – that will balance his humours.

■ ACTIVITY

Use the information from this section to make some important revision notes about Galen. Draw a diagram like the one below to organise your notes.

Background information about Galen

Existing ideas and methods followed by Galen

Galen

Galen's importance to the development of medicine

New ideas and methods used by Galen

New idea 2: the brain controls the body

> I proved that the brain controls speech. I also showed that the brain controls other parts of the body. Before me people thought that the heart controlled the body.

A famous experiment

Galen also visited Alexandria in Egypt where he was allowed to DISSECT human bodies. He learned a great deal about how the body works. However, dissection of humans was forbidden in Rome so he had to use pigs instead.

One day Galen did a famous experiment in front of an audience to prove his idea that the brain controls the body. He cut into a pig's neck and found the nerves. The pig squealed.

'Watch,' said Galen to his audience, 'I will cut this nerve but the pig will keep on squealing.'

He cut. The pig kept squealing. Galen cut another nerve. Again the pig squealed.

'Now,' said Galen, 'I will cut another nerve that controls the pig's voice. It will not squeal.'

Galen cut the nerve. The room was silent.

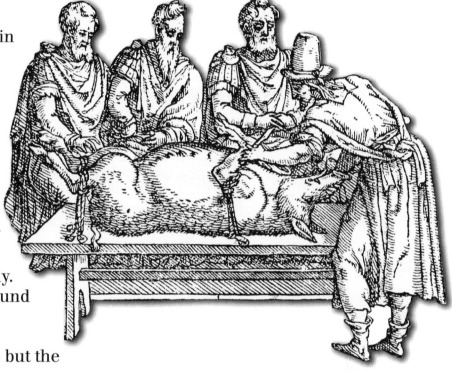

▼ **SOURCE 1** An illustration showing Galen's famous experiment. This was drawn hundreds of years later, in the Middle Ages

New idea 3: perfect design

> I also said that every organ in the body has a special role to play. It is as if the gods designed them all to fit together perfectly.

How important were Galen's ideas?

Galen's ideas and methods were extremely important. He had taken the best ideas of Hippocrates and the Greeks and combined them with his own work. Like Hippocrates, Galen also wrote down his ideas so that future doctors could learn from them. In fact, he wrote 60 books of medicine.

For the next 1500 years medical teaching was based on the ideas and methods described in Galen's books. Nobody dared to disagree with them. When Christianity became the main religion in western Europe, the Church supported Galen's ideas too. This was because they thought that Galen's ideas (see new idea 3) fitted in very well with the Christian belief that God created human beings.

1.7 *Review: From prehistory to the Romans*

Over the past chapter you have studied how medicine developed in Egypt, Greece and Rome. It's now time to compare those developments and to think about why they happened.

■ ACTIVITY 1

Look at Chart A and Chart B.

1 List three continuities in medicine. A continuity is something that stays the same.
2 Why did these things stay the same?
3 List three changes in medicine.
4 Why didn't these changes help people to live much longer?

Chart A

Healers and doctors

Some illnesses were healed by mothers and other women. Medicine men tried to cure more difficult illnesses.

Treatments

Herbs and other practical remedies were used for some problems. Magic charms and spells were used for others.

Medicine in prehistoric times

Explanations for disease

People thought that the gods and evil spirits caused diseases.

Chart B

Healers and doctors

Most illnesses were stilll treated by mothers and other women. But specialist doctors treated wealthy people or special groups such as soldiers.

Treatments

Herbs and magic charms and spells were still used. Other treatments were based on the theory of the four humours, such as bleeding, rest and exercise and the treatment of opposites.

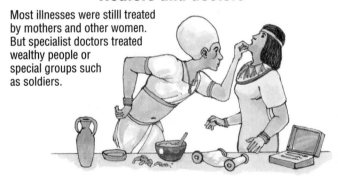

Medicine under the Egyptians, Greeks and Romans

Explanations for disease

Some people thought that the gods caused diseases. The Egyptians believed that blocked channels caused illness. The Greeks and the Romans developed the idea that people became ill when their humours were out of balance.

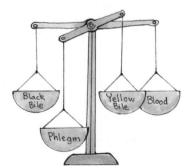

Preventing diseases spreading

The Romans developed public health schemes in towns. They provided fresh water supplies, sewers and baths.

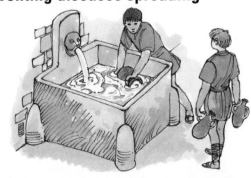

Who was the most important person in medicine?

■ ACTIVITY 2

5 Do you remember what Galen said on page 28? He said that he was the most important person in medical history. Now you have your chance to decide! Which of the people below do you think was the most important in medicine in Egypt, Greece and Rome? Write a paragraph giving two reasons for your choice.

I developed the theory of the four humours which was the basis for Galen's ideas. My ideas lasted for thousands of years.

I was one of the first doctors and thought of the first logical reasons for illness. The others would not have had their ideas if I had not been first.

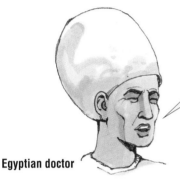

Egyptian doctor

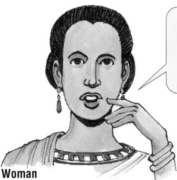

Hippocrates

Most illnesses are treated by mothers like me. We pass on herbal cures to our own children and grandchildren. They do far more good than all these fancy ideas.

Woman

I improved on Hippocrates' ideas and the important ideas in my books were used for over 1000 years – long after the engineer's sewers and pipelines were destroyed.

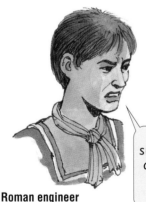

My sewers and clean water supplies saved many lives. It's a practical way of improving people's health, not just another fancy theory.

Roman engineer

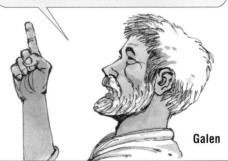

Galen

■ ACTIVITY 3

Important changes were made in medicine by the Egyptians, the Greeks and the Romans.

6 Explain the theory of the four humours.
7 Why did the Greeks make more advances in medicine than the Egyptians? Explain your answer.
8 Who made the more important contribution to the development of medicine, the Greeks or the Romans?

Why were there changes and continuities in medicine?

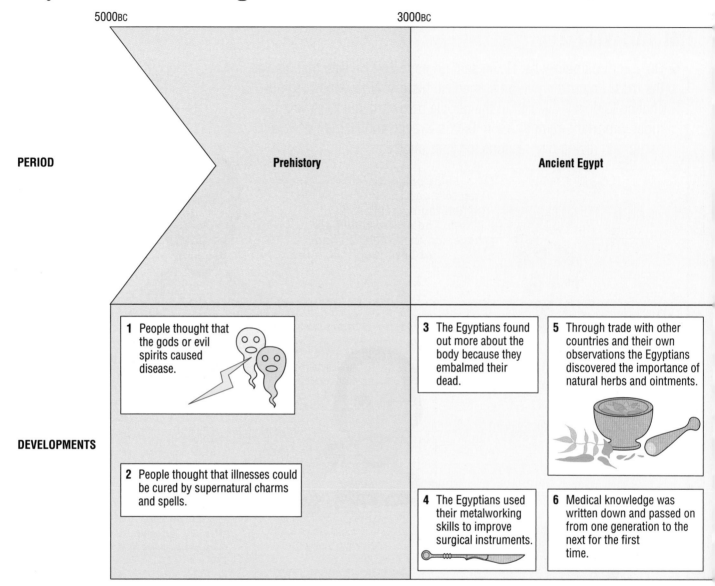

	5000BC	3000BC
PERIOD	**Prehistory**	**Ancient Egypt**

DEVELOPMENTS

1 People thought that the gods or evil spirits caused disease.

2 People thought that illnesses could be cured by supernatural charms and spells.

3 The Egyptians found out more about the body because they embalmed their dead.

4 The Egyptians used their metalworking skills to improve surgical instruments.

5 Through trade with other countries and their own observations the Egyptians discovered the importance of natural herbs and ointments.

6 Medical knowledge was written down and passed on from one generation to the next for the first time.

■ ACTIVITY

On the timeline are the main developments in medicine during the period you have been studying.
Now it's time to work out why some things in medicine changed and why some things stayed the same.
Here is a list of factors (reasons) why there were changes and continuities:

■ Attitudes and religious beliefs
■ War
■ Governments
■ Communications
■ Science and technology
■ Individual genius.

1 Make your own copy of the timeline.

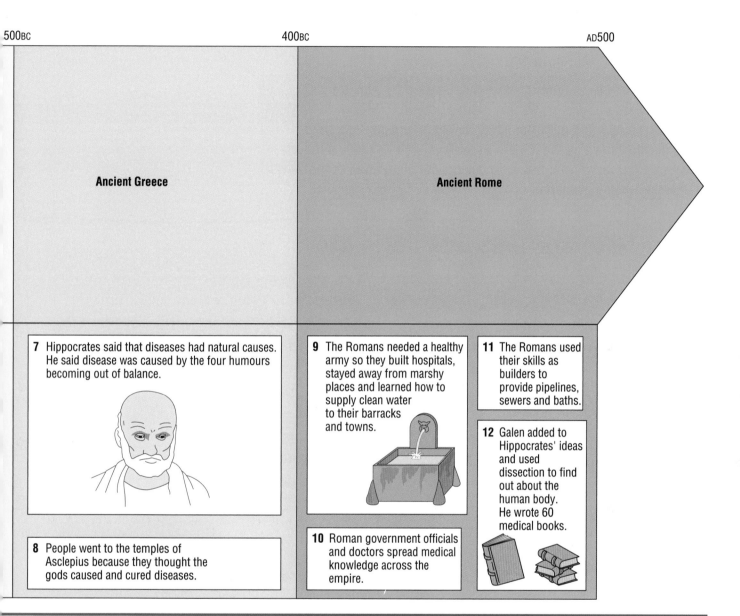

500BC · 400BC · AD500

Ancient Greece

Ancient Rome

7 Hippocrates said that diseases had natural causes. He said disease was caused by the four humours becoming out of balance.

8 People went to the temples of Asclepius because they thought the gods caused and cured diseases.

9 The Romans needed a healthy army so they built hospitals, stayed away from marshy places and learned how to supply clean water to their barracks and towns.

10 Roman government officials and doctors spread medical knowledge across the empire.

11 The Romans used their skills as builders to provide pipelines, sewers and baths.

12 Galen added to Hippocrates' ideas and used dissection to find out about the human body. He wrote 60 medical books.

2 Which factor fits which boxes on the timeline? Put a factor heading next to each box on your timeline. You can decide to give a box more than one factor heading.

3 Now draw a table like the one below and list the developments under each factor.

Attitudes and religious beliefs	War	Governments	Communications	Science and technology	Individual genius

4 Which of the factors was most important in changing medicine? Explain your choice.

5 Which of the factors was most important in stopping change in medicine? Explain your choice.

33

By AD400 the Roman empire was being invaded by warriors from northern Europe. As a result, the Roman army left Britain. In this chapter you will find out what happened to medicine next, in the long period known as the Middle Ages, from 400 to 1350. But first, what can you learn from this story about what happened to medicine when the Roman army left?

Escape into chaos and darkness

I am an old woman now but I can still remember the happy days when I was young. My father was a Roman officer who had lived in Britain for years. My mother was British. Father was not supposed to have a British wife and family but it didn't seem to matter – until the message came.

The message told the soldiers to return to Rome. Rome was being attacked by tribes from the north. Father said it was because the government in Rome was useless and had lost control. It was a terrible shock. There was no chance of our going to Rome with Father.

We stayed in Chester but the city began to change. There were no engineers like Father to solve the problems if something went wrong with the baths or the sewers. People stopped using the baths and wash-houses. Everywhere began to smell really dreadful. The aqueduct became fouled up and people just threw their garbage into the baths and sewers.

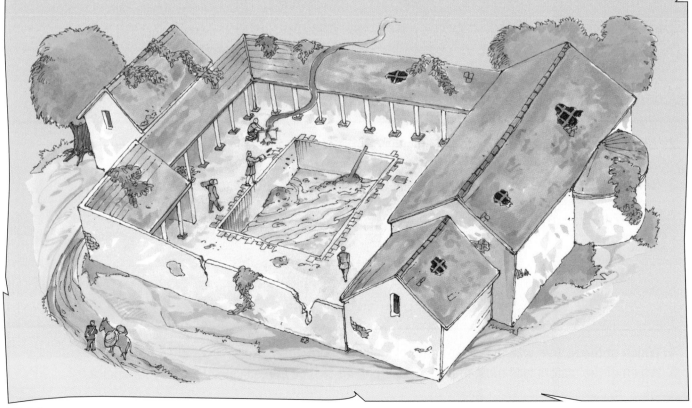

■ ACTIVITY

1 After you have read this story make three lists:
  a) all the ways the Romans had helped to improve medicine and health
  b) the problems or changes after the Romans left
  c) the continuities – things that stayed the same – after the Romans left.
2 What do you think were the TWO most important CHANGES?
3 Which do you think was the most important CONTINUITY?

4 Look at the list of factors below. Can you find any evidence in the story of any of these factors affecting medicine after the Romans left? Did they make medicine better or worse?

  ■ Attitudes and religious beliefs
  ■ War
  ■ Governments
  ■ Communications
  ■ Science and technology
  ■ Individual genius

Worse was to come. New tribes began to invade our area, looting and destroying. One day, my brother Quintus staggered home. He had been in a fight and was bleeding from a deep cut in his leg. Mother ran to Father's old house to get herbs and ointments but the store had been ransacked. Everything had been taken and all Father's medical books, including his precious copies of Galen's work, had been burnt. For a moment we panicked, then we remembered an old woman who made all kinds of medicines from herbs and plants. We had never needed her when Father was with us but now we had no choice.

She looked carefully at Quintus' leg and began collecting her medicines.

I remember she used some plantain, mixed with onion and garlic, as well as some other things. She pounded them together, then spread the mixture on the wound. For two weeks we went back every day so that she could check Quintus' leg and by the end of that time the wound was clean and healing nicely.

As soon as Quintus could walk again we gathered our belongings and set off for the marshland up river. Here we would be safe from the invaders from the west. We were joined by other families and we built ourselves houses among the marshes. Gradually, the chiefs of the invaders took over the area but they did not live in Chester. They were interested in war, not in building baths and aqueducts or reading books.

2.1 *Did medicine really get worse after the Romans?*

The Roman empire collapsed around AD400. Over the next four pages you will find out how this affected medicine and health.

With the Roman army gone there was no longer one government to control Britain. Instead there were many small kingdoms fighting each other for power and land. Some of these kingdoms were ruled by Saxon invaders.

Later, in the 800s and 900s, the Vikings invaded Britain. These new rulers were usually illiterate and so could not read the books left behind by the Romans. Some books were kept in MONASTERIES, including books by Galen and other doctors, but not many people read them.

The big idea in the Middle Ages was tradition – people did what they had always done and thought the old ways were the best. They did not want new ideas!

So the picture of medicine in the Middle Ages is like this:

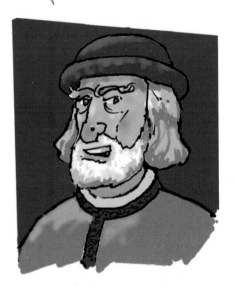

Our big idea is that we don't have new ideas!

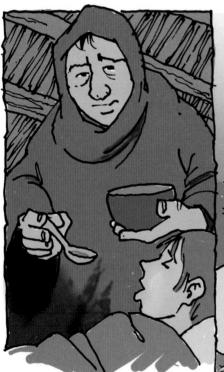

Most illnesses were treated by women at home with herbs and other remedies. If these did not work, people tried spells and prayers.

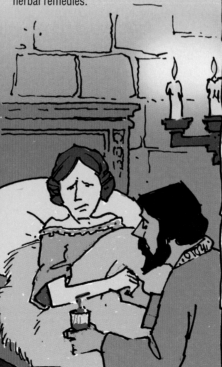

Rich people could pay a doctor to come and treat them if they were ill. Doctors used bleeding and other treatments based on the theory of the four humours as well as herbal remedies.

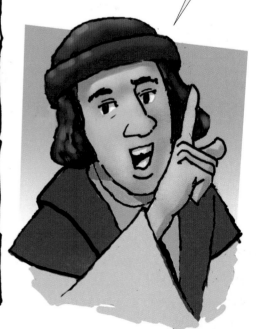

That's right. We must respect tradition. The old ideas are the right ideas.

Did herbal treatments work?

In the Middle Ages most illnesses were treated with herbal remedies. Doctors used them. Mothers and wise-women used them. Women healers treated far more people than doctors did and they knew a great deal about how to use herbs to treat illnesses.

Scientists today have analysed many herbal remedies. They have discovered that many herbs would have helped to cure illness. One example is a herb called plantain, which was used in 48 treatments in a MEDIEVAL medical book. Plantain is what is called an ANTIBIOTIC and would have helped in 25 of the 48 treatments listed. These included treatments for boils in the ear and for cuts and dog bites. Source 1 is another example.

■ DISCUSS

1 Why did the treatment in Source 1 work?
2 People in the Middle Ages did not know that the ingredients in Source 1 were antibiotics. Why did they use them?
3 Look at Source 2. Why did doctors bleed patients?
4 How does Source 2 show that there was some CONTINUITY in medicine after Roman times?

▼ **SOURCE 2** Bleeding was still one of the most common treatments. Doctors believed that bleeding restored the balance of the four humours in the body. It removed the excess blood that was making the patient ill

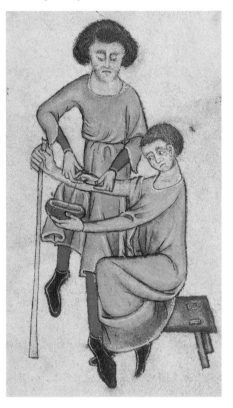

▼ **SOURCE 1** A medieval cure for a stye in the eye

The medieval remedy

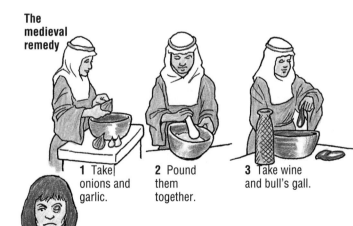

1 Take onions and garlic.
2 Pound them together.
3 Take wine and bull's gall.

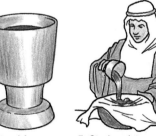

4 Stand for nine nights in a brass vessel.
5 Strain mixture through a cloth.

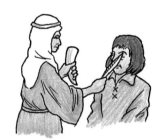

6 Apply to stye with a feather.

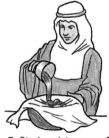

The modern verdict

Onion and garlic are antibiotics. They kill bacteria.

Bull's gall also attacks bacteria.

Wine contains acetic acid which reacts with copper in the brass vessel to form copper salts. These kill bacteria.

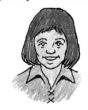

The result: a cure

Why did the Roman public health system collapse?

Before: the Roman public health system

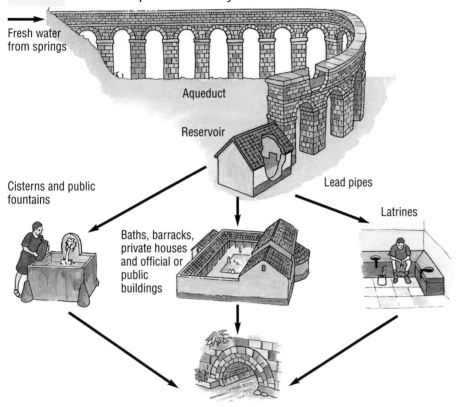

Fresh water from springs

Aqueduct

Reservoir

Cisterns and public fountains

Lead pipes

Latrines

Baths, barracks, private houses and official or public buildings

Sewers emptying into river

After: public health under the Saxons and Vikings

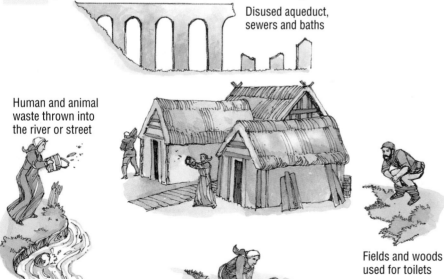

Disused aqueduct, sewers and baths

Human and animal waste thrown into the river or street

Fields and woods used for toilets

Drinking water taken from the river

■ ACTIVITY

The Roman public health system collapsed during the Saxon and Viking periods. The sewers and baths were still there but nobody used them. On this page you can see the differences between the two periods and opposite you can see some reasons why they were so different.

1 Look at the 'Before' and 'After' drawings on the left. List the changes in the public health system after the Romans left.

2 Which of these changes do you think had most effect on people's health? Explain your choice.

3 Look at the Roman senators above right. List:
   a) two reasons why the Romans needed a good public health system
   b) three reasons why the Romans were able to build a good public health system.

4 Look at what the Viking chieftains are saying bottom right. List:
   a) two reasons why the Vikings went to war
   b) two things the Vikings spent money on.

5 Write a paragraph to explain why you think the Roman public health system collapsed. Use your lists from questions 1–4 to help you write your answer.

Roman senators (politicians) discuss the public health system

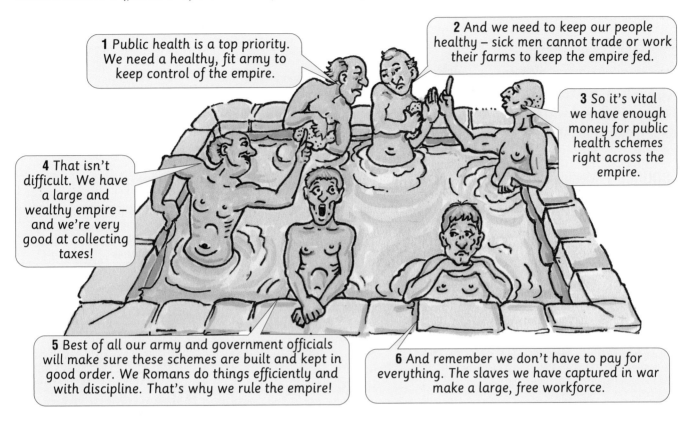

1 Public health is a top priority. We need a healthy, fit army to keep control of the empire.

2 And we need to keep our people healthy – sick men cannot trade or work their farms to keep the empire fed.

3 So it's vital we have enough money for public health schemes right across the empire.

4 That isn't difficult. We have a large and wealthy empire – and we're very good at collecting taxes!

5 Best of all our army and government officials will make sure these schemes are built and kept in good order. We Romans do things efficiently and with discipline. That's why we rule the empire!

6 And remember we don't have to pay for everything. The slaves we have captured in war make a large, free workforce.

Viking chieftains discuss their plans

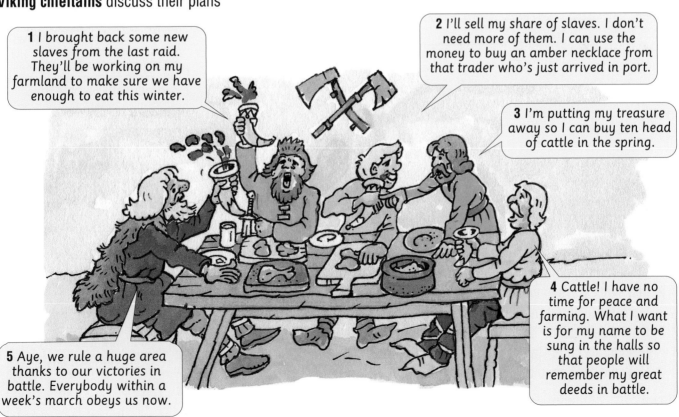

1 I brought back some new slaves from the last raid. They'll be working on my farmland to make sure we have enough to eat this winter.

2 I'll sell my share of slaves. I don't need more of them. I can use the money to buy an amber necklace from that trader who's just arrived in port.

3 I'm putting my treasure away so I can buy ten head of cattle in the spring.

4 Cattle! I have no time for peace and farming. What I want is for my name to be sung in the halls so that people will remember my great deeds in battle.

5 Aye, we rule a huge area thanks to our victories in battle. Everybody within a week's march obeys us now.

2.2 *Were Arab doctors better than European doctors?*

While the Saxons and Vikings were destroying what the Romans had made, the Arab world was not. In fact the Arabs preserved (looked after) and copied Greek and Roman books containing medical ideas. In this section you will be able to decide whether Arab doctors had better medical ideas than the European doctors.

▼ **SOURCE 1** Medicine in the Arab world and how it was connected to European medicine

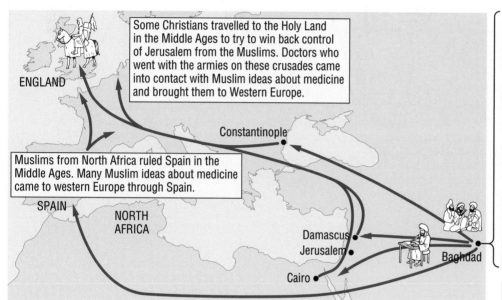

ENGLAND

Some Christians travelled to the Holy Land in the Middle Ages to try to win back control of Jerusalem from the Muslims. Doctors who went with the armies on these crusades came into contact with Muslim ideas about medicine and brought them to Western Europe.

Constantinople

Muslims from North Africa ruled Spain in the Middle Ages. Many Muslim ideas about medicine came to western Europe through Spain.

SPAIN

NORTH AFRICA

Damascus
Jerusalem
Cairo
Baghdad

Arab scholars translated the works of Galen and Hippocrates into Arabic and their work was read by medical students.

Arab doctors also increased their knowledge by learning from Indian and Persian doctors.

There were good libraries of medical works in cities such as Baghdad.

A Muslim physician called Avicenna wrote an important medical textbook. It was used throughout the Muslim world and in Europe for 600 years.

Arab religious law said that human bodies could not be dissected. Most Arab doctors believed that all the important information about how the body works had already been discovered anyway.

Caring for the sick is important in the Muslim faith. There were large hospitals in the major cities.

■ ACTIVITY

1 Look at the map in Source 1. How did the Muslim religion help to support medicine?

2 List three ways in which Arab doctors could learn more about medicine.

3 How did Avicenna learn about the ideas of Hippocrates and Galen?

4 How did Arab medical ideas affect European medicine?

5 Copy the table below. As you read pages 40–42, fill in your table with any evidence that supports either of the statements.

In some ways Arab medicine was BETTER than European medicine	In some ways Arab medicine was SIMILAR to European medicine

Story 1: A woman with fever

Now for a different kind of evidence about Arab medicine. Source 2 is a story written by an Arab nobleman called Usamah. He lived near Jerusalem over 800 years ago in the 1100s. At that time, many Europeans lived around Jerusalem. Usamah had European friends and he saw European doctors as well as Arab doctors at work. This story is about an Arab doctor called Thabit.

▼ SOURCE 2

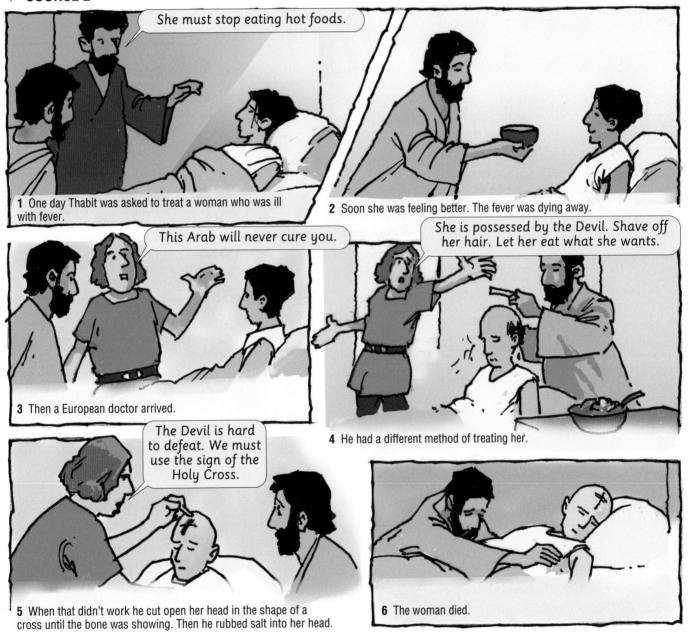

1 One day Thabit was asked to treat a woman who was ill with fever.

2 Soon she was feeling better. The fever was dying away.

3 Then a European doctor arrived.

4 He had a different method of treating her.

5 When that didn't work he cut open her head in the shape of a cross until the bone was showing. Then he rubbed salt into her head.

6 The woman died.

■ DISCUSS

6 What methods were used to heal the woman by:
   a) Thabit, the Arab doctor?
   b) the European doctor?

7 What caused the woman's illness, according to:
   a) Thabit, the Arab doctor?
   b) the European doctor?

Story 2: Sir Bernard's foot

▼ **SOURCE 3**

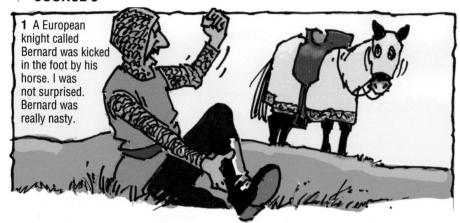

1 A European knight called Bernard was kicked in the foot by his horse. I was not surprised. Bernard was really nasty.

2 Bernard's foot was badly cut and would not heal. His doctors could not help him.

I don't know how to treat his wound.

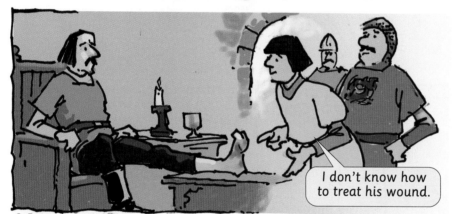

3 Then another European doctor came to see him.

This needs washing regularly in vinegar. That will heal the wound.

4 He was right. Soon the wound healed and Bernard was back to normal – fighting anyone he met!

If you need some more evidence to help you to decide whether Arab medicine was better than European medicine, read this second story by Usamah (Source 3).

■ DISCUSS

1 What does Source 3 tell you about the skills of European doctors?
2 Why do you think the injury healed? (You'll have to think! The story does not tell you.)
3 Do you think that Usamah gives us reliable evidence about doctors and medicine?

You should have learned quite a lot about Arab and European doctors from Usamah's stories.

Many Arab doctors were very skilful. Medical understanding and skills were often better in Arabia than in Europe. However, that does not mean that all Arab doctors were better than all European doctors. There were some good European doctors, like the one in the second story, who used successful treatments and cures.

2.3 *Why was change in medicine very slow between 1000 and 1350?*

By AD1000 Europe was recovering from centuries of war and bad government. Medicine began to improve slowly. You are going to examine why the changes happened but also why they were so slow. This section will also be good for practising source handling skills which you will need for your exam.

Communications
Merchants from different countries began trading with each other more and more. At the same time they collected ideas and books about medicine from the Muslims in Arabia. Some of these were the ideas of Galen, but they also learned some new ideas from Arab doctors.

Governments
There were laws to force towns and cities to clean up. However, there were no police to enforce the laws and there was no money from the king to pay for improvements.

Factors explaining CHANGE and CONTINUITY in the Middle Ages

War
Armies took trained doctors to war with them where they gained experience as surgeons on the battlefield. However, because kings spent a lot of money on war, they did not spend it on public health schemes, like water pipes and sewers.

Attitudes and religious beliefs
The Christian Church set up universities where doctors could be trained. It also built hospitals for the sick. Some of the Church's monasteries contained books by Greek and Roman writers, such as Hippocrates and Galen. These books were copied and sent to other monasteries.

However, the universities did not teach the doctors to look for new ideas. They taught that Galen's ideas were correct and that there was no need to do more research into the causes of illness or treatments.

■ ACTIVITY

1 Draw a table like the one below. Fill it in using Sources 1–7 on pages 44–48.

Source	Which factor is the source telling you about?	Did this factor keep medicine the same, help it to change – or a little of both?

2 Take a large sheet of paper – at least A3 size. Divide it up into three sections.
  a) In section 1 describe the factors that caused slow change in medicine.
  b) In section 2 describe the factors that prevented changes in medicine.
  c) In section 3 explain why there was more continuity than change in medicine.

▼ **SOURCE 1** A teacher watching over a dissection. The teacher read out to the students parts of Galen's books. At the same time the body was dissected to show the students what Galen meant.

The Church allowed only one dead body a year to be used, so the students spent most of their time reading Galen's books. The teacher thought that Galen was right about everything

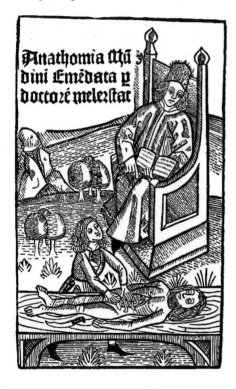

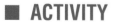

▼ **SOURCE 2** Theodoric of Lucca, an army surgeon, 1214. Theodoric is describing his experiences as an army surgeon during the Crusades

... every day we see new instruments and new methods being invented by clever and ingenious surgeons.

He disagreed with other army surgeons:

They teach that pus should be generated in wounds. There could be no greater error than this. For it does nothing else but hinder the work of nature, prolong the disease, prevent healing and the closing up of wounds. ... My father used to heal almost every kind of wound with wine alone and he produced the most beautiful healing without any ointments.

Most surgeons disagreed with Theodoric because his ideas were different from Galen's. So they did not use wine to clean wounds and their patients died from infections.

▼ **SOURCE 3** This chart gave details about when each part of the body was affected by the planets and stars. If the stars told the surgeon not to open wounds or bleed the patient in that area then he would not do so, because he thought the patient would die. Charts like this, known as the 'Zodiac man', were much in use

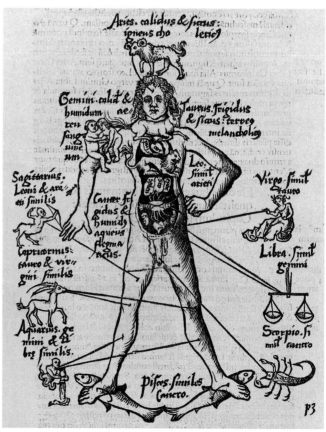

■ ACTIVITY

1 What does Source 3 tell you about ideas about the causes of disease in the Middle Ages?

2 Does this source prove that no one tried to improve medicine in the Middle Ages? Use all the sources and your background knowledge to explain your answer.

Find…

3 Find … in Source 4:

- nuns sewing the dead bodies into bags. How would this prevent disease from spreading?
- nuns feeding the sick. How would this help their patients?
- an altar with a statue of the crucified Christ. What can you learn from its position?

▼ **SOURCE 4** The Hôtel Dieu – the largest medieval hospital in Paris, built by the Christian Church and opened in 1452. From 1100 onwards, the Christian Church learned from the Muslims, who built many hospitals because helping the poor and sick is very important to the Islamic faith. In hospitals the main treatments were prayer, food, rest and herbal medicines. People with infectious diseases were not admitted to hospitals. Most patients were just old and poor and unable to look after themselves

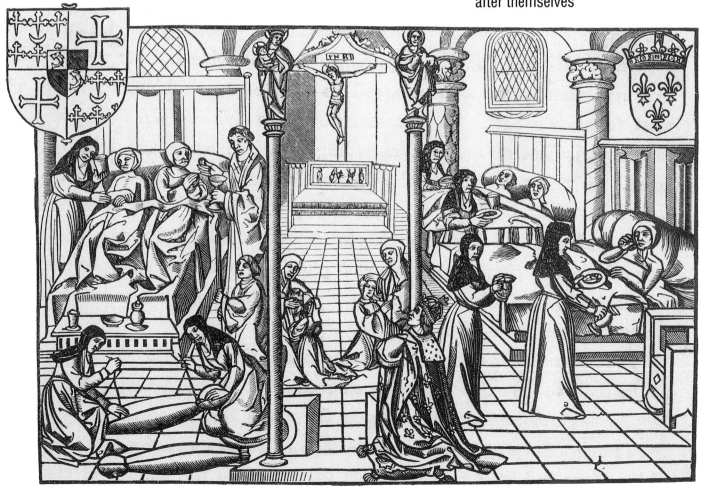

▼ **SOURCE 5** Public health in London in the fourteenth century

1 There were open sewers carrying refuse to the rivers.

2 1343 – butchers were ordered to use a segregated area for butchering animals.

3 By the 1380s there were at least thirteen common privies (public toilets) in the city. One on Temple Bridge was built over the Thames.

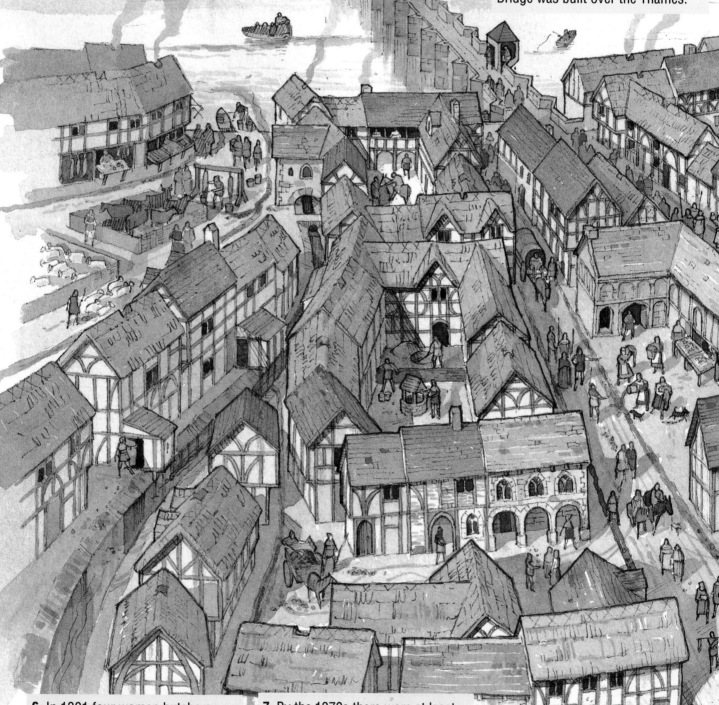

6 In 1301 four women butchers were caught throwing rotten blood and offal (animal intestines) into the street.

7 By the 1370s there were at least twelve teams of rakers with horses and carts, removing dung from the streets.

8 In 1364 two women were arrested for throwing rubbish into the street.

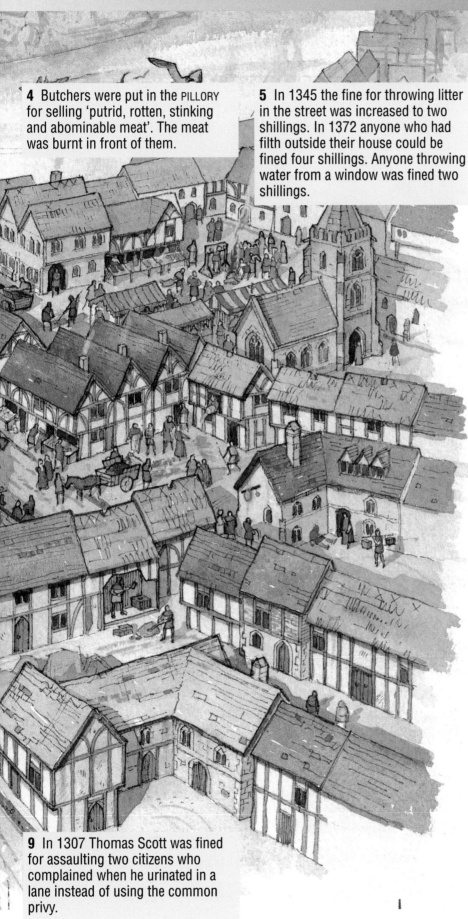

4 Butchers were put in the PILLORY for selling 'putrid, rotten, stinking and abominable meat'. The meat was burnt in front of them.

5 In 1345 the fine for throwing litter in the street was increased to two shillings. In 1372 anyone who had filth outside their house could be fined four shillings. Anyone throwing water from a window was fined two shillings.

9 In 1307 Thomas Scott was fined for assaulting two citizens who complained when he urinated in a lane instead of using the common privy.

■ **ACTIVITY**

1 The events described in the nine boxes are hidden in the picture. Can you find them?

■ **DISCUSS**

2 Look at Sources 5 and 6. Choose three of the measures taken and explain how you think they would have made London a healthier place.

3 Do Sources 5 and 6 prove that people cared whether their towns were clean? Explain your answer.

▼ **SOURCE 6** A letter written in 1349 by King Edward III to the Lord Mayor of London

To the Lord Mayor of London. Order to cause the human faeces (excrement) *and other filth lying in the streets and lanes in the city and its suburbs to be removed with all speed and the city to be cleaned as it used to be.*

The King has learned how the city and suburbs are so foul with filth from the houses that the air is infected and the city poisoned.

SOURCE 7 A diagram of the water supply to Canterbury Cathedral and monastery. Monks in monasteries taught people that fresh water was vital to good health. Here, water was piped to the kitchen, washrooms, brewery, bakery and fishponds. Waste water was also recycled to flush the latrines. The Church and its monasteries were very wealthy. They had the money to pay for pipes, fresh water supplies and sewers. This was the nearest anyone came in the Middle Ages to the Roman public health schemes

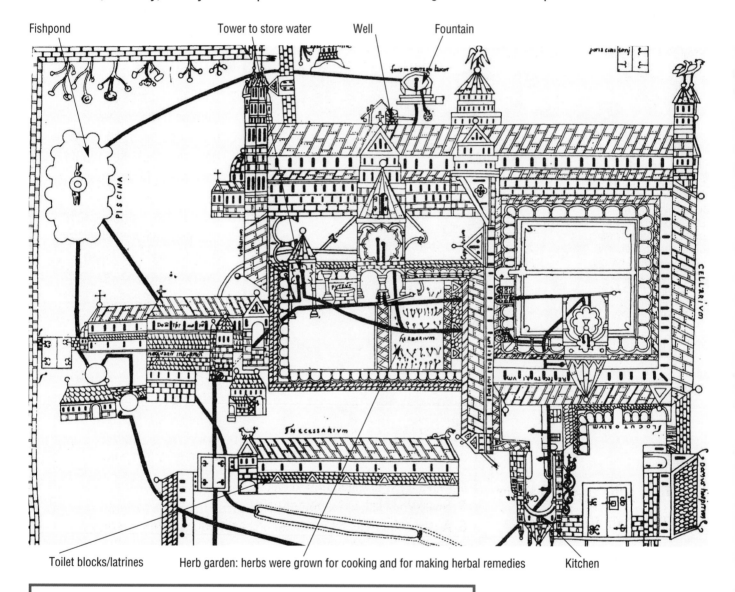

Fishpond   Tower to store water   Well   Fountain

Toilet blocks/latrines   Herb garden: herbs were grown for cooking and for making herbal remedies   Kitchen

■ ACTIVITY 1

1 Look at Source 7. Make a list of all the different ways in which monastic life kept its monks fit and healthy.
2 What does Source 7 tell you about ideas about public health in the Middle Ages?
3 Does Source 7 prove that people in the Middle Ages worked hard to improve public health? Use the source and your background knowledge to explain your answer.

Medicine in the Middle Ages: a summary

Treatments
Most people used herbal remedies. Many of these worked but, if not, there was not much anyone could do – except pray! Surgeons could do simple operations, but there were no safe ANAESTHETICS (pain killers).

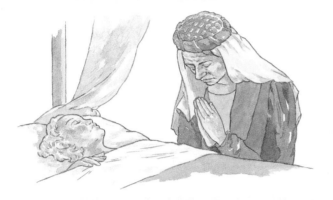

Preventing diseases spreading
Governments made some efforts to keep towns clean. However, they did not have the money or the workforce to build pipes for clean water or for sewers, as the Romans did. More importantly, kings were usually too busy with other things, such as wars or keeping law and order, to spend time and money on public health.

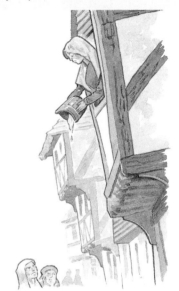

Explanations of disease
Nobody understood the true causes of disease. Doctors believed that people became sick when their humours were out of balance. Many ordinary people believed sickness was a punishment from God, or the work of the Devil.

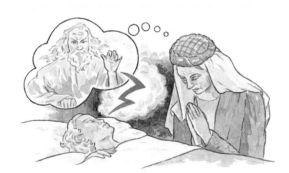

■ **ACTIVITY 2**

Work in pairs. Go back in time to interview a medieval doctor.

4 Make a list of questions to ask him.
5 Swap your list with another pair.
6 Answer the other pair's questions as if you were the medieval doctor.

Galen – still the greatest doctor of them all!

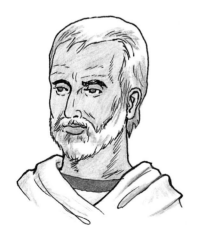

Why was change in medicine very slow between 1000 and 1350?

By 1350 there were some doctors, such as Theodoric (Source 2), who were starting to look for new 'big ideas'. However, most doctors in the Middle Ages did not try to make new discoveries because they believed Galen had all the answers.

2.4 *The Black Death – a case study in medieval medicine*

In 1348 a terrible disease spread across much of Asia and Europe. In England it was called the Black Death. Over the next four pages you will study the Black Death to find out how people explained it at the time. At the end you will decide whether these explanations of disease in 1350 are similar to or different from the explanations used by the ancient Egyptians, Greeks and Romans. You will also practise some important exam skills.

Throughout the history of medicine some people have looked for natural explanations of disease. For example Hippocrates and Galen said that illness was caused when the four humours became unbalanced. This was a natural explanation. However they could not explain or cure all illnesses, so many people continued to believe that gods or evil spirits caused illness. This was a supernatural explanation.

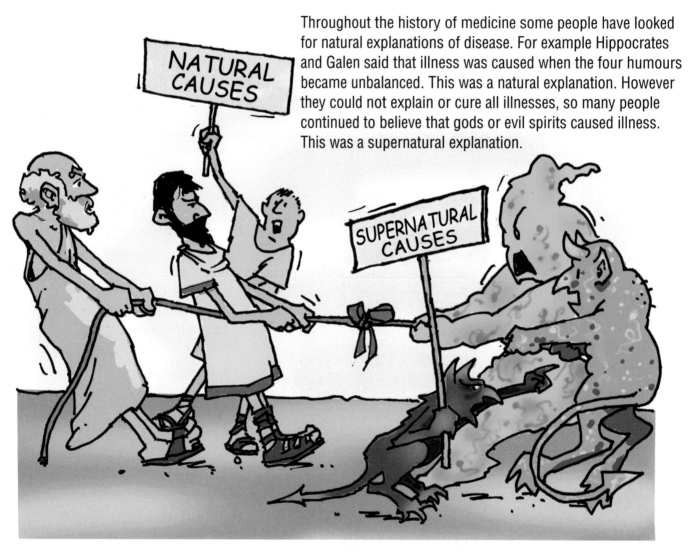

The question you can now investigate is:

Had ideas about the causes of disease changed by the end of the Middle Ages?

What was the Black Death?

In 1348, a ship brought the Black Death to England. Source 1 describes its arrival. Even more people died than the monk thought. Over 40 per cent of the population died during the plague. The Black Death killed rich and poor alike, and it killed swiftly and painfully. The dead were quickly buried in large communal graves.

▼ **SOURCE 1** Written by a monk in Wiltshire in 1350

… the cruel pestilence [plague] arrived on the south coast of England at Melcombe in Dorset. Travelling all over the country it killed people in Dorset, Devon and Somerset. Next it travelled northwards, leaving not a city, a town or a village without killing most or all of the people so that over England a fifth of the men, women and children were carried to burial.

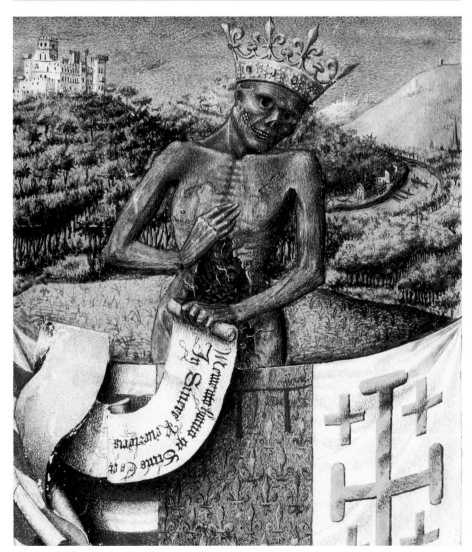

We now know that the Black Death included two kinds of plague:

■ **Bubonic plague**, in which painful swelling (buboes) appeared in people's armpits and groin. They got a high fever and headache. They became unconscious and died a few days later in dreadful pain. This type of plague was spread by fleas.

■ **Pneumonic plague**, which attacked people's lungs. They coughed up blood and died very quickly. This form of plague was spread by people breathing or coughing germs on to one another. People in the Middle Ages did not know this. Over the page you can find out how they explained the plague.

◄ **SOURCE 2** King Death, a painting from a French prayer book

■ **DISCUSS**

Look at Source 2. Why do you think death is shown as a king?

What did people in the Middle Ages think caused the Black Death?

■ ACTIVITY 1

1 On these pages you can see six sources and six cartoons. These show different explanations for the Black Death. Match up the sources to the correct cartoons.

2 Copy this table and then fill it in, showing which sources give natural and which give supernatural explanations for the Black Death.

Source number	Natural explanations	Supernatural explanations

▼ SOURCE 3 Guy de Chauliac, a famous doctor in the 1300s

The particular cause of the disease in each person was the state of the body – bad digestion, weakness and blockage, and for this reason people died.

▼ SOURCE 4 Guy de Chauliac, a famous doctor in the 1300s

The general cause was the close position of the three great planets, Saturn, Jupiter and Mars. Such a coming together of planets is always a sign of wonderful, terrible or violent things to come.

▼ SOURCE 5 A letter to the Bishop of London, 1348

Terrible is God towards the sons of men ... He often allows plagues, miserable famines, conflicts, wars and other forms of suffering, and uses them to terrify and torment men and so drive out their sins.

▼ SOURCE 6 From an account of the plague by a French doctor, 1349

This epidemic kills almost instantly, as soon as the airy spirit leaving the eyes of the sick man has struck the eye of a healthy bystander looking at him, for then the poisonous nature passes from one eye to the other.

▼ SOURCE 7 From the writings of John of Burgundy, 1365

Many people have been killed, especially those stuffed full of evil humours. As Galen says in his book on fevers, the body does not become sick unless it already contains evil humours.

▼ SOURCE 8 From an account by a fifteenth-century Swedish bishop

Sometimes the pestilence comes from a privy [toilet] next to a chamber or any other particular thing which corrupts the air ... sometimes it comes of dead carrion or the corruption of standing waters in ditches.

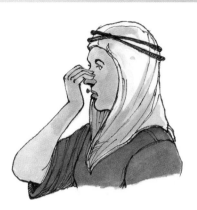

A The body's humours are out of balance

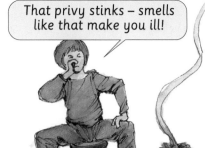

That privy stinks – smells like that make you ill!

B Common sense reasons

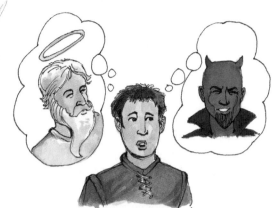

C God's punishment

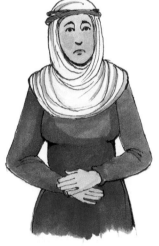

D Blocked digestive system

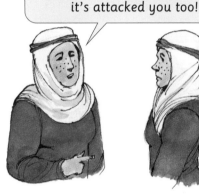

Something attacked me but I couldn't see what it was ... and it's attacked you too!

E Invisible spirits in the air

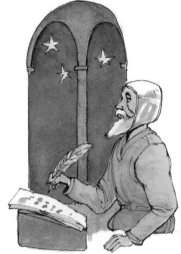

F The effects of the planets

■ DISCUSS

As you discuss the following questions, write down any important points made by people in your class.

3 Were ideas about the causes of the Black Death the same as the ideas about disease in ancient times (look back to pages 9 and 16)?

4 Why do you think people in 1350 did not understand what caused the Black Death?

■ ACTIVITY 2

5 Use the information on pages 36–53, and any notes that you have made, to help you to write a short essay. Here is the title:

'Ideas about the causes of disease were the same in the Middle Ages as they had been in ancient times.' Do you agree?

This question asks you write about both the similarities AND the differences. Then you must decide whether there were more similarities than differences.

■ In paragraph 1 explain what ideas people had about the causes of disease in the ancient world.

■ In paragraph 2 give one or more examples of medieval ideas about the causes of disease that were THE SAME as in Greek and Roman times.

■ In paragraph 3 give one or more examples of medieval ideas about the causes of disease that were DIFFERENT from Greek and Roman times.

■ In your final paragraph write a conclusion stating whether you agree or disagree with the main question. Show that your conclusion is backed up by the evidence you have provided.

CHAPTER 3 *Renaissance medicine 1350–1750*

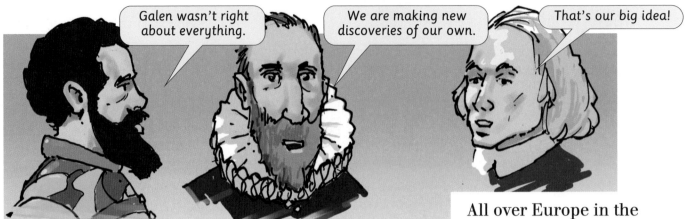

Andreas Vesalius

Galen wasn't right about everything.

We are making new discoveries of our own.

That's our big idea!

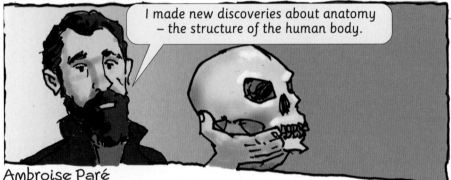

Ambroise Paré

I made new discoveries about anatomy – the structure of the human body.

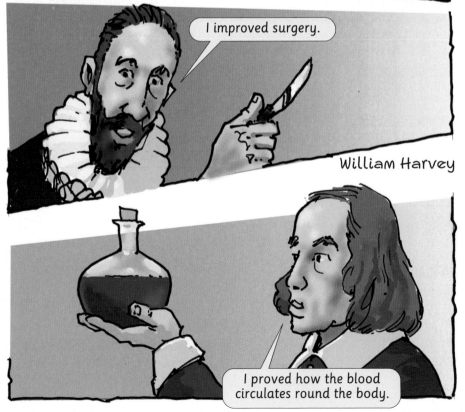

William Harvey

I improved surgery.

I proved how the blood circulates round the body.

All over Europe in the fifteenth century, educated people were questioning old ideas.

For example, Galileo carefully observed the sun and the stars and then he said that he disagreed with the traditional teaching that the sun moved around the earth. He said the earth moved around the sun. He used scientific methods – observation and experiment – to make new discoveries.

The same happened in medicine. In the Middle Ages most doctors had accepted that Greek and Roman writers like Galen were right about everything. Now, doctors had a new big idea. They challenged Galen and made new discoveries of their own.

Another important development was the invention of the printing press. This helped new ideas to spread more quickly.

This period is called the Renaissance, which means 'rebirth'.

At the same time there were great changes in art.

▶ **SOURCE 1** Giotto's painting of the *Madonna with Child*, 1310

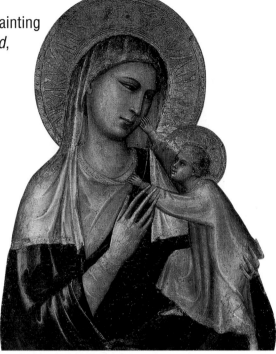

■ **DISCUSS**

1 Medieval artists had not tried to draw 'real people'. Renaissance artists such as Botticelli studied the human body carefully and tried to paint exactly what they saw. What clues in Source 1 show that Giotto did not study the human body to paint his pictures?
2 What clues in Source 2 show that Botticelli studied the human body?
3 Can you work out how artists who studied the human body closely could help doctors?

▼ **SOURCE 2** Botticelli's *Birth of Venus*, 1486

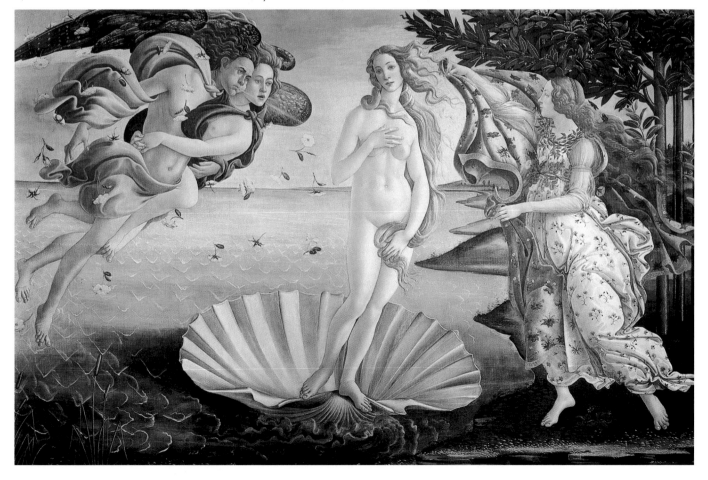

3.1 *Three great discoveries!*

Over the next six pages you are going to find out about the Medical Renaissance. You will read short biographies of three of the most important individuals from that time and draw up a table to compare them.

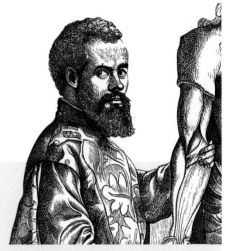

Andreas Vesalius

Born in Brussels in 1514. Studied medicine in Paris and Italy where he met artists who were studying skeletons and dissecting bodies to make their paintings more realistic. He became professor of surgery at Padua in Italy. Wrote *The Fabric of the Human Body* (published 1543) with detailed illustrations of the human body. Died in 1564.

Specialism
Anatomy

Importance
Before Vesalius: doctors believed that the books of Galen and other ancient doctors were completely accurate. They thought there was nothing more to learn.

After Vesalius: Vesalius showed that some of Galen's ideas about anatomy were wrong. He thought this was because Galen had had to dissect animals instead of humans. He said it was vital for doctors to dissect human bodies to find out exactly how the body works. He said doctors needed to test Galen's ideas, instead of accepting them without question.

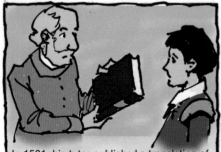

In 1531, his tutor published a translation of Galen's works on anatomy. Vesalius was fascinated.

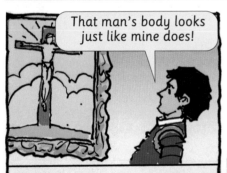

Vesalius was born in 1514, when artists like Michelangelo were painting humans who looked real!

> That man's body looks just like mine does!

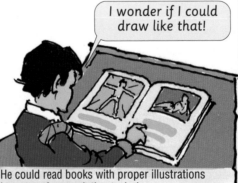

He could read books with proper illustrations because of new printing techniques.

> I wonder if I could draw like that!

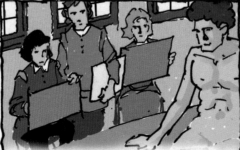

After three years in Paris Vesalius moved to Padua in Italy. He met artists who were dissecting and drawing human bodies.

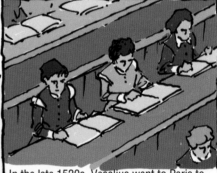

In the late 1520s, Vesalius went to Paris to study medicine.

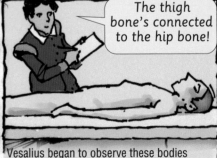

Vesalius began to observe these bodies scientifically. He drew and labelled each separate part. He began to make connections.

> The thigh bone's connected to the hip bone!

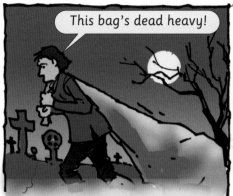

He needed more and more bodies, so that he could develop his scientific methods. He began to steal bodies from graves or gallows.

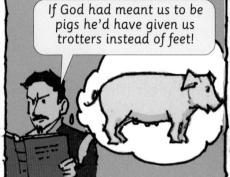

Vesalius discovered that some of Galen's ideas about anatomy were wrong. He realised that this was because Galen had had to dissect pigs and monkeys, not humans.

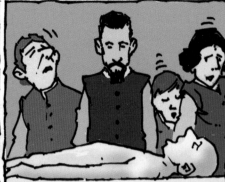

Vesalius realised that his students needed to learn about anatomy from human corpses, not animals.

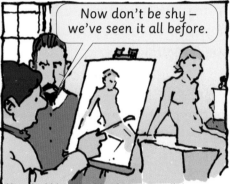

He asked his artist friends to draw all the different parts of the human body. Vesalius was now Professor of Surgery at Padua University, so people were willing to help him.

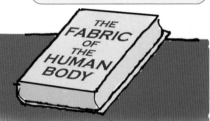

He put the artists' drawings together in a book called *The Fabric of the Human Body*, which was published in 1543. Vesalius used the best artists and the best printing techniques for his book.

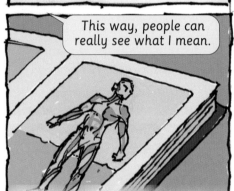

He always used modern technology. He used the most modern scalpels for his dissections. He wrote about what he had found when dissecting the bodies and used the drawings to help him to explain things properly.

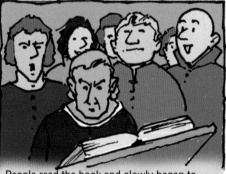

People read the book and slowly began to realise that Galen hadn't got everything right.

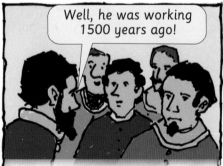

Later on, Vesalius said that Galen's ideas about the heart were wrong too.

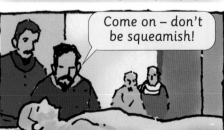

This book changed people's knowledge about the human body. Vesalius said that doctors could only find out the truth by dissecting and studying human bodies themselves, not just by reading Galen.

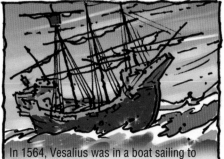

In 1564, Vesalius was in a boat sailing to Cyprus. A storm blew up, the boat was wrecked and Vesalius drowned.

■ ACTIVITY

1 Read the information box and the story strip on these pages.
2 Now copy and complete this table using a full sentence for each cell.

	Vesalius
Discoveries	
How he used scientific methods	
Importance in history of medicine	

Ambroise Paré

Born in France in 1510. He was apprenticed to his brother, a barber surgeon, and then became a surgeon at the Hôtel Dieu in Paris (see page 45). In 1536 he became an army surgeon and spent twenty years on campaigns, treating sword and gunshot wounds. He wrote *Works on Surgery*, published in 1575. He died in 1590.

Specialism
Surgery

Importance
Before Paré: wounds were treated by pouring boiling oil on them. Surgeons stopped wounds from bleeding by sealing them with hot irons.

After Paré: Paré discovered that wounds healed more quickly if oil was not used. He used his own ointment. He stopped using hot irons to seal wounds. Instead he used silk threads to tie the ends of the blood vessels.

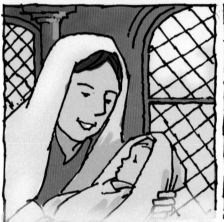

Ambroise Paré was born in France in 1510.

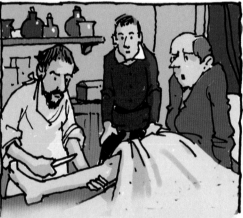

He liked watching his older brother, who was a barber surgeon, operate on his patients.

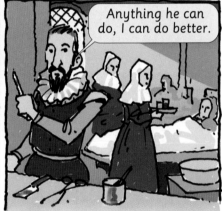

Anything he can do, I can do better.

When he was nineteen, Paré decided to become a surgeon too. He got a job in Paris at a famous hospital called the Hôtel Dieu.

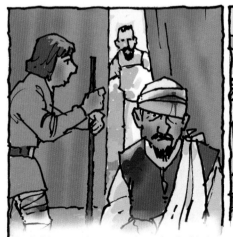

Paré did not earn very much, so he decided to join the army as a surgeon.

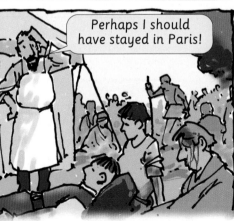

Perhaps I should have stayed in Paris!

He went off to war. One day, the fighting was really bad. Hundreds of soldiers had gunshot wounds.

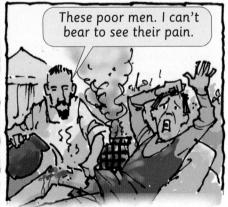

These poor men. I can't bear to see their pain.

Paré and the other surgeons treated wounds as normal, by pouring boiling oil on them. The men screamed in agony as the oil CAUTERISED their wounds.

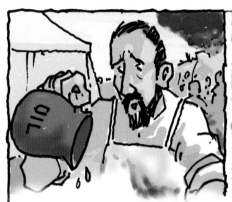

Paré ran out of oil. He still had many patients to look after. Then he remembered what the Romans had used.

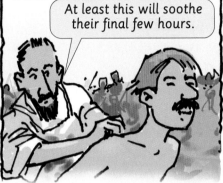

At least this will soothe their final few hours.

Paré quickly made an ointment as the Romans used to do, with egg yolks, oil of roses and turpentine. He spread the ointment on to the gunshot wounds.

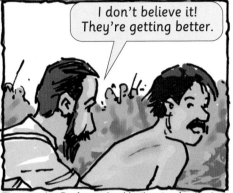

I don't believe it! They're getting better.

The next day Paré examined both sets of patients. The men who had been treated with boiling oil were still in agony, the men who had been treated with ointment were calm and rested.

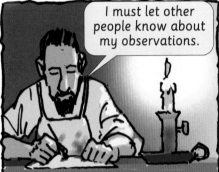

I must let other people know about my observations.

Paré decided never to use the old treatments again. He had carefully and scientifically observed his patients and written down what he saw.

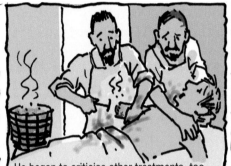

He began to criticise other treatments, too, such as the one used after AMPUTATING limbs. The old way was to press a hot iron against the stump of the limb to cauterise it and stop the bleeding. Patients often died in agony!

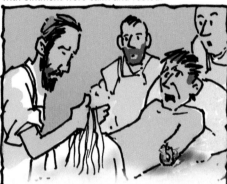

Paré now tried a new way. He tied silk thread around each of the blood vessels. This was called a LIGATURE and stopped the bleeding.

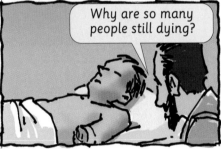

Why are so many people still dying?

This method was better than the old method. But people still got infections because Paré did not use clean thread. He didn't know that germs caused disease.

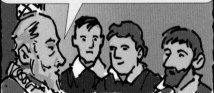

Have respect for the old ways but believe in your own ideas too!

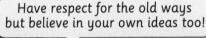

As Paré became famous, people began to listen to him. He was important in medicine because he challenged the old ways of doing things. This gave other doctors confidence to try new methods too.

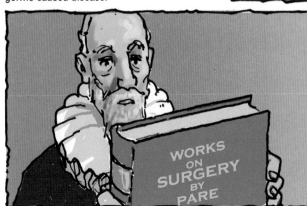

When Paré retired from the army he became a surgeon to the French kings. In 1575 he wrote a book called *Works on Surgery*. It was translated into many languages. Doctors all over Europe read it and copied Paré's ideas.

■ ACTIVITY

1 Read the information box and the story strip on these pages.

2 Now add another column to your chart from page 57.

	Paré
Discoveries	
How he used scientific methods	
Importance in history of medicine	

William Harvey

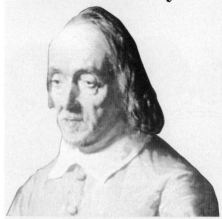

Born in Kent in 1578. Studied medicine at Cambridge and Padua. Worked as a doctor in London. In 1628 he published *An Anatomical Account of the Motion of the Heart and Blood in Animals*. He died in 1657.

Specialism
The circulation of the blood.

Importance
Before Harvey: many doctors still believed Galen's idea that new blood was constantly being made in the liver to replace blood that was burnt up in the body, in the same way that wood is burnt up in a fire. Some doctors thought this idea was wrong but no one had been able to find out exactly how the blood did move around the body.

After Harvey: Harvey showed that blood flows around the body and that it is carried away from the heart in arteries and returns to the heart in veins. He proved that blood is not burnt up and replaced with new blood. The heart pumps blood round and round the body.

▼ **SOURCE 1** How the heart pumps blood around the body

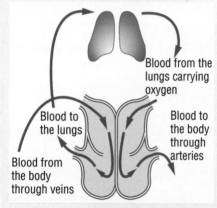

Blood from the lungs carrying oxygen

Blood to the lungs

Blood to the body through arteries

Blood from the body through veins

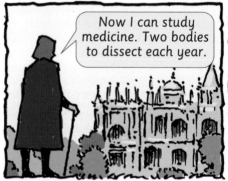

At the age of sixteen, Harvey went to Cambridge University.

Now I can study medicine. Two bodies to dissect each year.

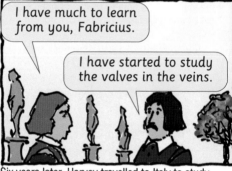

I have much to learn from you, Fabricius.

I have started to study the valves in the veins.

Six years later, Harvey travelled to Italy to study with famous doctors such as Hieronymus Fabricius. He completed his studies when he was 24.

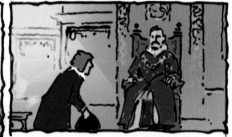

He became very successful and returned to London. In 1607 he was made a Fellow of the Royal College of Physicians. Then he was put in charge of St Bartholomew's Hospital. Finally, Harvey became physician to King James I.

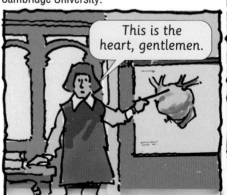

This is the heart, gentlemen.

In 1615, Harvey began lecturing on anatomy to the public.

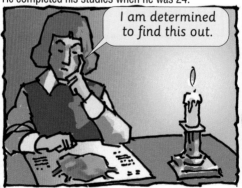

I am determined to find this out.

He could not work out how the blood kept moving around the body.

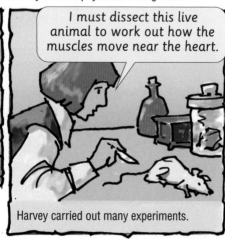

I must dissect this live animal to work out how the muscles move near the heart.

Harvey carried out many experiments.

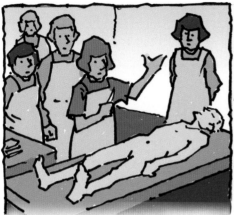

He dissected human bodies so that he could observe the heart more closely.

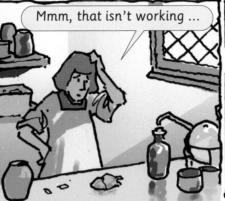

Mmm, that isn't working …

He experimented by trying to pump liquids past the valves of the heart into the veins, but could not do so.

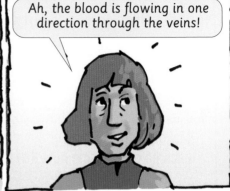

Ah, the blood is flowing in one direction through the veins!

He pushed thin rods down the veins and worked out that blood flowed in a one-way system around the body.

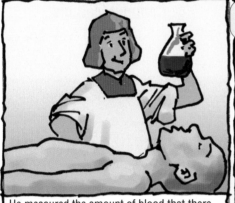

He measured the amount of blood that there was in the body.

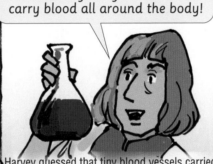

It's amazing! Tiny blood vessels carry blood all around the body!

Harvey guessed that tiny blood vessels carried blood around the body, even though he could not see them because microscopes at that time were not good enough.

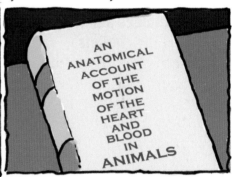

AN ANATOMICAL ACCOUNT OF THE MOTION OF THE HEART AND BLOOD IN ANIMALS

In 1628, Harvey published his findings in a book called *An Anatomical Account of the Motion of the Heart and Blood in Animals*. He had proved that the heart pumped blood around the body.

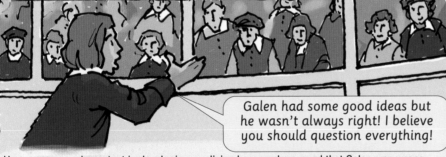

Galen had some good ideas but he wasn't always right! I believe you should question everything!

Harvey was very important in developing medicine because he proved that Galen was wrong about anatomy. He changed the way people thought and gave other doctors confidence to experiment too.

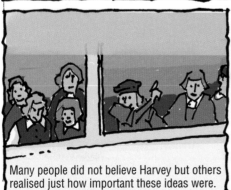

Many people did not believe Harvey but others realised just how important these ideas were.

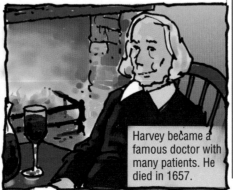

Harvey became a famous doctor with many patients. He died in 1657.

■ ACTIVITY

1 Read the information box and story strip on these pages.

2 Now add another column to your chart from page 57.

	Harvey
Discoveries	
How he used scientific methods	
Importance in history of medicine	

Why did the three men make these discoveries?

Now it's time to work out why these discoveries were made.

■ ACTIVITY

1 The diagram below shows you that four factors helped Vesalius. Make your own copy of the diagram and write one sentence in each box explaining how that factor helped Vesalius.

Attitudes and religious beliefs

Communications

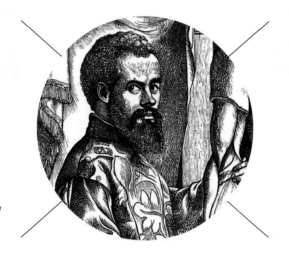

Science and technology

Individual genius

2 Now draw your own diagrams for Paré and Harvey BUT this time you will have to work out which factors to put in the boxes and how many boxes there should be. Choose the factors from the list below.

Factors that have helped to change medicine
- Attitudes and religious beliefs
- War
- Governments
- Communications
- Science and technology
- Individual genius

Enquiry and challenges to tradition

1350

1750

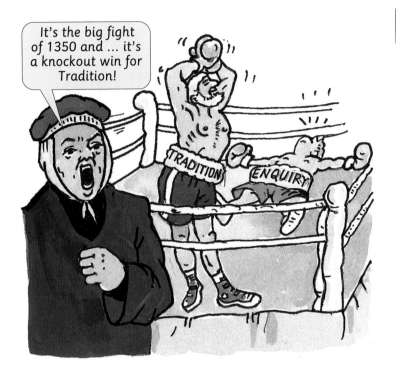

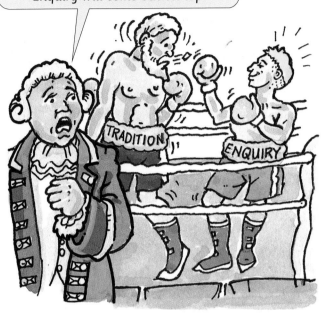

LED TO

Discoveries by:

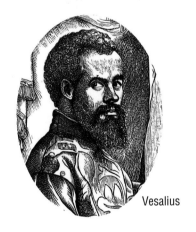

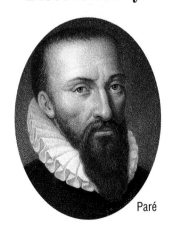

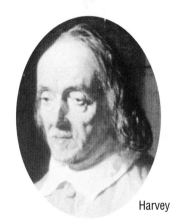

Vesalius

Paré

Harvey

HELPED BY

Social changes

- Better education
- The invention of printing
- Improved technology, e.g. better microscopes

3.2 Why weren't people any healthier by 1750?

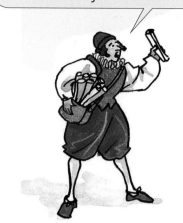

Read all about it! Great medical discoveries! Nobody getting any healthier for centuries!

> **Medical knowledge may have been improving but that did not mean that people were healthier or living longer lives. That sounds odd but now you can work out why.**

The discoveries by Vesalius, Paré and Harvey did not make people live longer because the discoveries were no help for the everyday diseases and illnesses that killed most people – for example, diarrhoea from infected water; plague; SMALLPOX; influenza; blood poisoning; or infections in childbirth.

Their discoveries did *not* improve understanding of what caused these diseases and illnesses ...

When plague struck London in 1660 people still had the same explanations of disease as they had when the Black

Death struck 300 years earlier. Vesalius, Paré and Harvey had no effect on the understanding of disease.

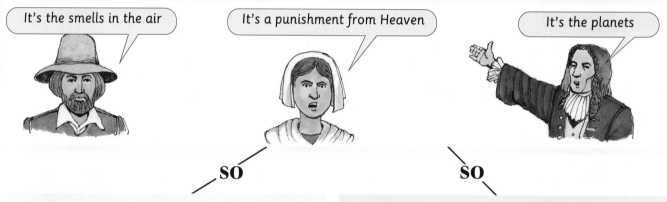

It's the smells in the air

It's a punishment from Heaven

It's the planets

SO   **SO**

... their discoveries did *not* affect treatment or provide cures for disease

People kept on using the old treatments for the next few centuries. They could not think of anything else to do. So when the plague came they bled themselves, or mixed up a herbal remedy or carried posies of flowers to ward off the bad smells. Vesalius, Paré and Harvey had no effect on treatments for disease.

... their discoveries did *not* persuade governments to improve public health

Clean water and good sewers were the main things that would make people healthier and live longer, but

- governments still did not think it was their job to provide clean water and did not have the skills or the money to do this
- people still did not understand how important clean water was to health. Vesalius, Paré and Harvey had no effect on attitudes to public health.

▼ **SOURCE 1** Doctors applying leeches in the late 1700s. This was a way of bleeding patients – the leeches sucked out blood

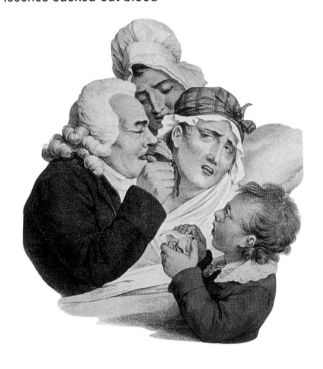

■ **DISCUSS**

1 How does Source 1 show you that Galen's ideas were still being used?
2 What was the great step forward in the Medical Renaissance?

So, you are probably wondering, if Vesalius, Paré and Harvey did not help with these things, why are they important? There are two reasons:

Their attitudes

Vesalius's and Harvey's discoveries about anatomy and the circulation of the blood proved that Greek and Roman thinking *could* be wrong. Their attitude was to challenge old ideas, not just to accept them. They showed that careful dissection and experiment could lead the way to new understanding. This inspired other scientists and doctors to make new discoveries too.

Their methods

They used scientific approaches. They observed. They experimented. They watched what happened. They changed their methods if they did not work. This scientific method did eventually begin to have an effect on medicine. For example, one doctor, Edward Jenner in 1798, used careful observation and experiment to discover a way of preventing the deadly killer disease smallpox. You will find out about Jenner on pages 72–73. People like Vesalius, Paré and Harvey led the way in using scientific methods.

■ **ACTIVITY**

3 Harvey is looking for an assistant to help him in his research. List two qualities he would most look for.
4 'The Medical Renaissance did not help people to live any longer or help to cure any illnesses so it was not important.' Write a paragraph to explain why this statement is wrong.

In the next chapter you are going to study how, eventually, these attitudes and methods began to have an effect where it really mattered – on ordinary people's health.

The period of time you are about to study is known as the Industrial Revolution. It is called this because there was a REVOLUTION – a big change – in the way people worked. Before 1750, most of the work was done in the countryside, on farms or in small towns and villages. After 1750, great new technological inventions meant that huge factories were put up, canals, roads and railways were built and people moved from the countryside to the big cities to find jobs.

The Industrial Revolution, like most revolutions, had its good points and its bad points. As far as medicine goes, it was good that there were new machines, new technology and new ideas to help doctors and scientists. It was bad that people moved from the fresh air of the countryside to dirty, cramped and overcrowded SLUMS in the cities where diseases spread very easily.

■ ACTIVITY

1 Why do you think living conditions like those in Source 1 were so dangerous to health?

▼ **SOURCE 1** An engraving of terraced houses in London by Gustav Doré, 1872. Industrial towns were full of these grim terraces. Houses were crammed together close to factories and workshops because, until the later 1800s, people had to walk to work – there was no transport. Some older houses were built without sewers, fresh water or toilets. People collected water from pipes in the streets. Refuse piled up in gutters

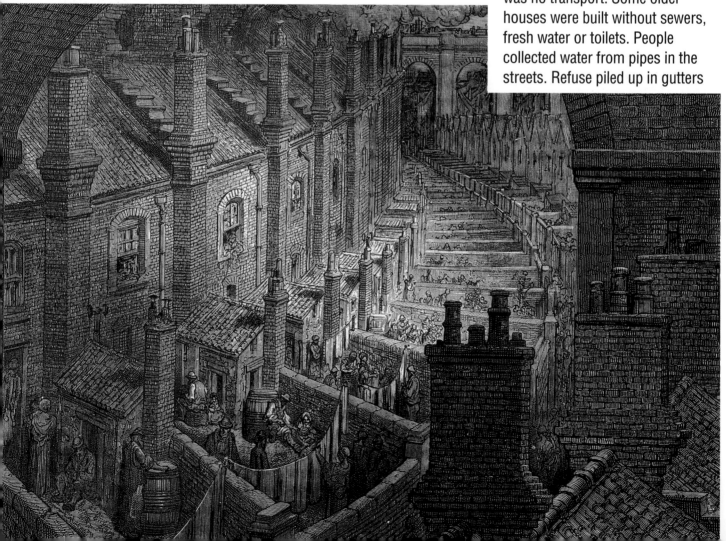

This period is so important in medical history that there are TWO big ideas, not just one!

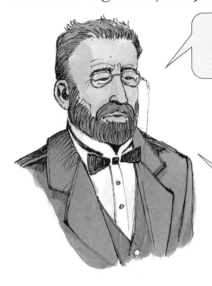

Big idea 1

Now we know what really causes disease – germs!

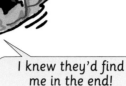

I knew they'd find me in the end!

Big idea 2

Now governments spend lots of money on providing sewers and clean water supplies to stop diseases spreading.

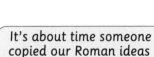

It's about time someone copied our Roman ideas on public health.

■ DISCUSS

2 Can you spot the link between the two big ideas?

3 How do you think these changes were linked to the big idea in the last chapter?

▼ **SOURCE 2** Factors leading to change in medicine, 1750–1900

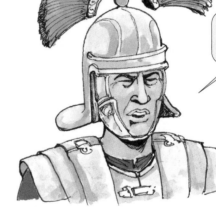

The rapid growth of towns increased the dangers of epidemic disease and made people realise that they must work together to improve health.

People's attitudes to poverty and sickness changed. The wealthy wanted reforms that would improve everyone's health.

Factors leading to change in medicine, 1750–1900

Government's attitude changed. It began to force local councils to improve public health by providing sewers and clean water.

There were many **huge engineering projects**, such as the building of canals and railways. These developed the skills and experience that could be used in public health schemes.

Scientific knowledge and technology improved rapidly.

4.1 *The main changes 1750–1900*

Between 1750 and 1900 many discoveries were made which had a great impact on medicine and health. Here they are – your task is to make them into a timeline.

Timeline: developments and discoveries in medicine during the nineteenth century

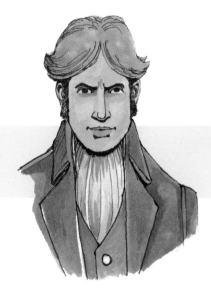

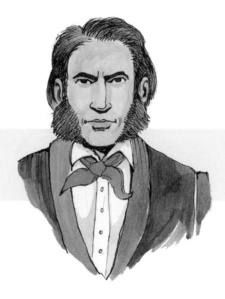

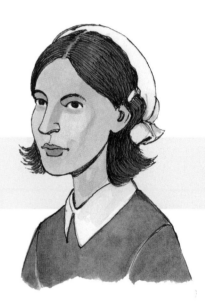

1798 Edward Jenner developed a VACCINE for smallpox.

1847 James Simpson discovered anaesthetics.

1850 Florence Nightingale developed new attitudes towards health and cleanliness.

Consequences of these developments and discoveries

1 At long last people realised that evil spirits, bad humours or bad smells did not cause disease. They could look for more suitable treatments.

2 Doctors were able to keep wounds clean and clear of infection.

3 Patients slept when they were operated on. They no longer suffered terrible agonies that often killed them through shock!

■ ACTIVITY

Between 1750 and 1900 discoveries were made that led to more real improvements in medicine than ever before.

1 Match each development or discovery in the top row of the timeline to the correct consequence or effect in the bottom row.
2 Redraw the timeline in your own book, showing the correct consequence for each development or discovery.

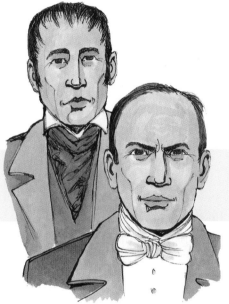

1854 Edwin Chadwick and John Snow realised that there was a link between dirt and disease.

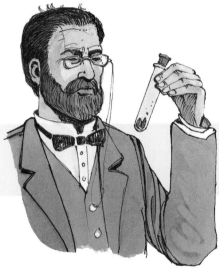

1861 Louis Pasteur discovered germs.

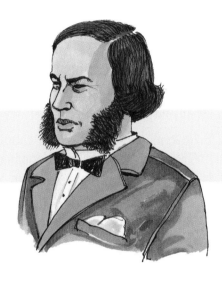

1867 Joseph Lister discovered ANTISEPTICS.

4 A way had been found of preventing the spread of infectious disease.

5 Filthy slums were cleaned up. People now had clean drinking water. Sewers were built underground.

6 Hospital patients were more likely to survive because wards were kept clean and nurses were better trained.

4.2 *'Medical Marvels of the Millennium'*

On pages 72–84 you are going to look at some of the key individuals who were behind the discoveries in your timeline. Your task is to choose the four people who most deserve a place in the 'Medical Marvels of the Millennium Hall of Fame'.

■ ACTIVITY

Medical Marvels of the Millennium

You are a member of a panel of judges who must decide which famous people will have their portrait hung in the nineteenth century 'Medical Marvels of the Millennium Hall of Fame'. The seven people in your timeline are the candidates. You must use the selection criteria (reasons for your choice) listed in the table below to select only **four** out of the seven.

1 Read all of the information about the seven people on pages 72–84.
2 Complete the activities connected to them.
3 Copy out and complete a score card like the one below for each person (in pencil first of all).
4 Now compare them, and make up your own mind, using the scores you have given them on the score cards.
5 When you have chosen the four for the Millennium Hall of Fame, write some notes to go with each portrait. These should explain why the person is so important in the history of medicine. They should be no more than one side of A4.

Name of Medical Marvel:				
Selection criteria	Totally agree 3 points	Agree almost completely 2 points	Agree 1 point	Disagree 0 point
1 Made an important new discovery or introduced a new method of treatment that no one else had ever thought of.				
2 Used scientific methods to get evidence for the discovery or method of treatment.				
3 Saved the lives of millions of people who would have died without this discovery or method of treatment.				
4 The new discovery or method of treatment has stood the test of time and is still used today.				
5 The new discovery or method of treatment led to other people making more improvements in the same area of medicine.				

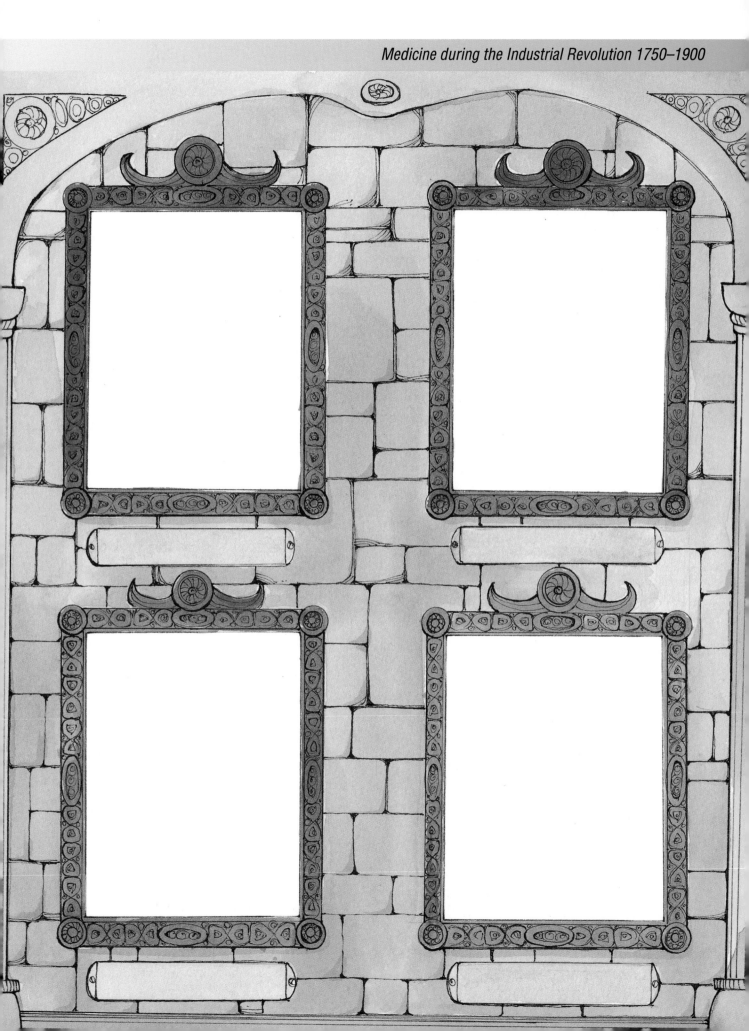

Medical Marvels Candidate 1: Edward Jenner

Between 1721 and 1798 two different people found out how to stop people catching smallpox. This was a dreadful disease that killed many people. Those who were lucky enough to survive were left with terrible scars all over their bodies.

Discovery 1: Lady Mary Wortley Montagu and inoculation

The first discovery was made by Lady Mary Wortley Montagu in 1721. When she was travelling in Turkey, she noticed that the people there had a very good method of preventing the spread of smallpox. They put the pus from someone with a smallpox scab on to an open cut in the skin of someone without smallpox. This gave that person a mild dose of the disease – gave them IMMUNITY (see Source 1) – and stopped them from getting a full-blown attack.

Lady Montagu decided to INOCULATE her own children in the same way. They survived the next smallpox epidemic. In England people respected Lady Mary. Within ten years, doctors were copying her method.

Discovery 2: Edward Jenner and vaccination

Edward Jenner was a doctor in Gloucestershire. Local people believed that people did not catch smallpox if they had already had cowpox. This was a mild form of the disease that dairymaids often got. Jenner wondered whether he could use cowpox as a method of preventing smallpox. He decided to **experiment** (see Source 2).

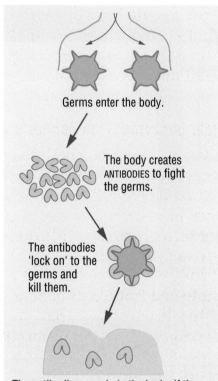

▼ **SOURCE 1** How immunity works

Germs enter the body.

The body creates ANTIBODIES to fight the germs.

The antibodies 'lock on' to the germs and kill them.

The antibodies remain in the body. If the same type of germs enter the body in future the antibodies are ready to fight them straightaway.

▼ **SOURCE 2** Extracts from Dr Jenner's casebook, 1798

Case 16
Sarah Nelmes, a dairy maid, was infected with cowpox from her master's cows. A large sore and the usual symptoms were produced.

Case 17 James Phipps
I selected a healthy boy about eight years old. The matter (pus) was taken from the cowpox sore on the hand of Sarah Nelmes and was inserted on 14 May 1796 into the boy by two cuts each about half an inch long. On the seventh day he complained of uneasiness, on the ninth he became a little chilly, lost his appetite and had a slight headache, but on the following day he was perfectly well.

Then he was inoculated with smallpox matter (pus), but no disease followed.

Jenner did the same experiment 23 times with different people. After this he had definite proof. He wrote that *'the cowpox protects the human constitution* [body] *from the infection of smallpox'*. He published his findings in 1798. Jenner called this new method of preventing smallpox 'vaccination', after the Latin word for a cow – *vacca*.

How important was Jenner's work?

Edward Jenner's work was extremely important. He did not know exactly why his vaccine worked, but he had used careful observation and experiment to achieve his result. This meant that he had learned from Vesalius, Paré and Harvey. Hundreds of thousands of people were protected from getting smallpox as a result of his discovery. In 1852, more than 50 years after Jenner's discovery, vaccination was made compulsory. You can see the results in Source 3.

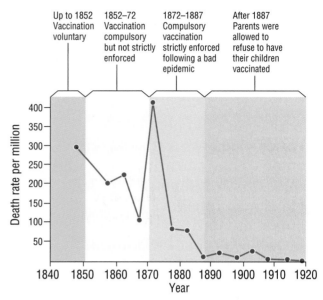

SOURCE 3 Graph showing deaths from smallpox

Jenner was also very important because he was the first person ever to IMMUNISE people against disease. Fifty years later, Jenner's methods were to be copied by other famous scientists such as Louis Pasteur and Robert Koch.

■ DISCUSS

1 What was Jenner's discovery?
2 How was Jenner helped by developments during the Medical Renaissance (see pages 54–55)?
3 Look at Source 3.
   a) What does this tell you about the impact of Jenner's discovery?
   b) Why do you think vaccination was not compulsory for many years? (You will find out more about this over the page.)
4 Look at the diagram on the right. Do you think Lady Montagu should be added to it? Explain your reasons why or why not.

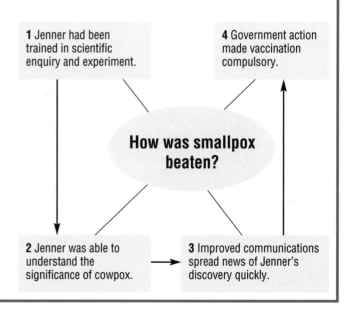

How was smallpox beaten?

1 Jenner had been trained in scientific enquiry and experiment.

4 Government action made vaccination compulsory.

2 Jenner was able to understand the significance of cowpox.

3 Improved communications spread news of Jenner's discovery quickly.

How did people react to Jenner's discovery?

You might think that people would have been delighted about Jenner's discovery, and would have wanted to be vaccinated straightaway. In fact, many people were opposed to Jenner's new method. There were many reasons why people were against vaccination:

- Some people did not like anything new and they thought Jenner's idea was very odd. They kept using traditional remedies like smearing boiled turnips on their feet.
- Some people did not accept Jenner's evidence. They said it was unbelievable that a disease from cows could protect humans.
- Doctors who made money out of giving inoculations (Lady Montagu's way) did not want to lose income.
- Vaccination was seen as dangerous. Some doctors mixed up their vaccines. Others used infected needles!

▼ **SOURCE 4** 'The cowpock – or – the Wonderful Effects of the New Inoculation!', a cartoon by James Gillray, published by the Anti-Vaccine Society in 1802

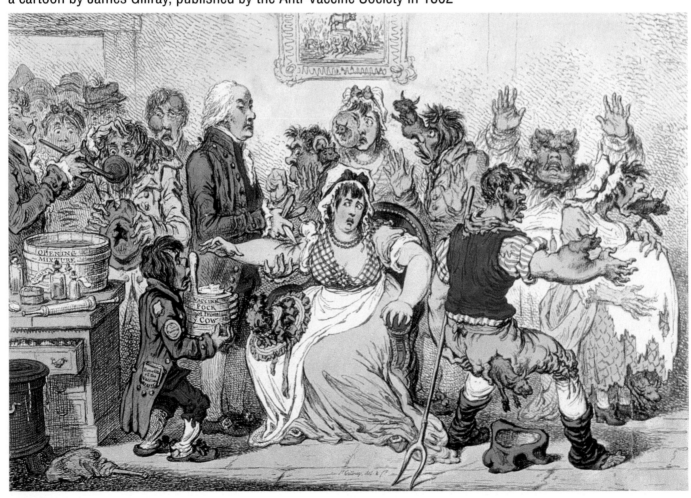

■ ACTIVITY 1

1 What reasons did James Gillray have for drawing the cartoon in Source 4?

2 Look again at Source 4. List all of the clues that tell you that the cartoonist was *against* vaccination.

3 Now look at Source 5. List all of the clues that tell you that the cartoonist was *for* vaccination.

4 Write a paragraph explaining why there was so much opposition to vaccination in the nineteenth century.

■ ACTIVITY 2

5 Fill out a score card (see page 70) for Edward Jenner.

▼ **SOURCE 5** 'The curse of humankind', a cartoon by George Cruikshank, 1808

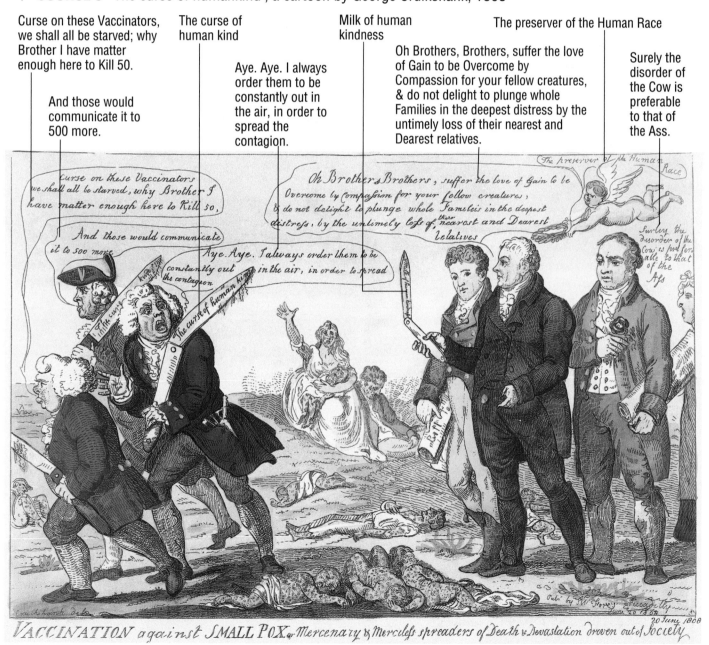

Curse on these Vaccinators, we shall all be starved; why Brother I have matter enough here to Kill 50.

And those would communicate it to 500 more.

The curse of human kind

Aye. Aye. I always order them to be constantly out in the air, in order to spread the contagion.

Milk of human kindness

Oh Brothers, Brothers, suffer the love of Gain to be Overcome by Compassion for your fellow creatures, & do not delight to plunge whole Families in the deepest distress by the untimely loss of their nearest and Dearest relatives.

The preserver of the Human Race

Surely the disorder of the Cow is preferable to that of the Ass.

VACCINATION against SMALL POX, or Mercenary & Merciless spreaders of Death & Devastation driven out of Society

Medical Marvels Candidate 2: James Simpson

Your second candidate discovered how to make operations less painful. Here is a description of an operation *before* James Simpson made his discovery:

▼ **SOURCE 6** The novelist Fanny Burney's account of her operation in 1811

When the dreadful steel was plunged into the breast – cutting through veins – arteries – flesh – nerves – I began a scream that lasted during the whole time of the incision – so excruciating was the agony. When the wound was made, and the instrument was withdrawn, the pain seemed undiminished, for the air that rushed into those delicate parts felt like a mass of sharp daggers that were tearing at the edge of the wound ...

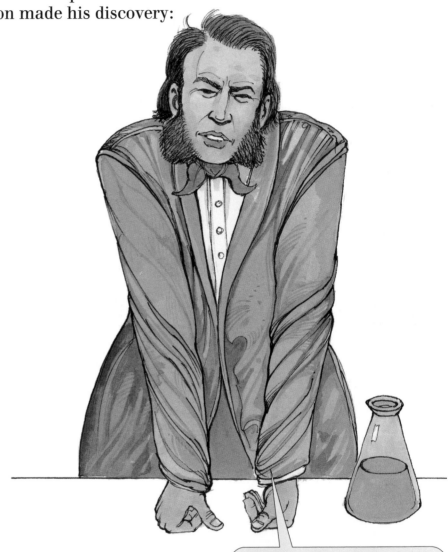

1 In 1847 I was the Professor of Midwifery at Edinburgh University. It made me so angry seeing how much suffering women went through in childbirth. I watched other operations too. They were dreadful. I was determined to do something to help these people.

■ DISCUSS

1 Read Source 6. How do you think Simpson would have felt if he had watched an operation like this?
2 Read what Simpson says about his discovery. Was it just chance that Simpson made his discovery or were there other reasons too?
3 Why did some doctors oppose anaesthetics?
4 How did Queen Victoria help to end opposition to anaesthetics?

■ ACTIVITY

5 Fill out a score card for James Simpson.

2 One day I was with friends. We decided on an experiment. Although other people had tried laughing gas and ether to reduce their patients' pain no one had thought of the chemical I wanted to use!

I poured some CHLOROFORM into three glasses. Before sitting down to supper we all inhaled the fluid and were 'under the table' in a minute or two. My wife was terrified.

We felt no pain even though our heads must have hit the chairs and table. I realised that I had discovered an excellent anaesthetic.

If we had felt no pain, then people could be given operations and feel no pain too. Surgeons could also take more time and care when operating on their patients. I soon used it to help relieve women's pain during childbirth and I wrote articles about it so other doctors could copy my ideas.

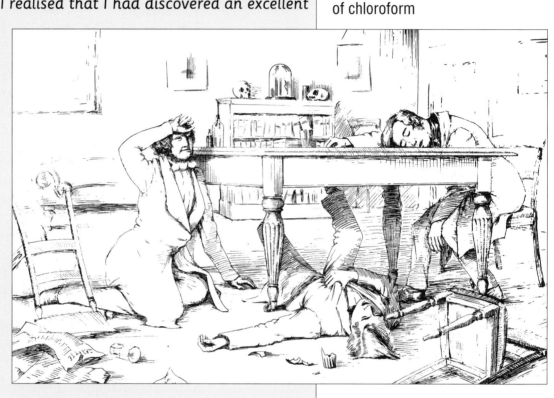

▼ **SOURCE 7** Simpson and friends recovering from the effects of chloroform

3 At first, many doctors who should have known better were against my discovery. They said that pain had been invented by God. They even said that the pain of childbirth made women more religious and improved their moral character. I could not agree with these people.

However, I accept that there were some problems. Some surgeons used too much chloroform. This led to patients dying.

Other surgeons got carried away when they realised their patients could not feel anything. They cut too many blood vessels and their patients died of infection or bled to death.

It has taken ten years for my great discovery to be recognised properly. However, now that our great Queen Victoria has used chloroform when giving birth in 1857, I know that my place in the Medical Marvels of the Millennium Hall of Fame is assured!

Medical Marvels Candidates 3 and 4: Edwin Chadwick and John Snow

1 My name is Edwin Chadwick. I work for the government.

In 1834, I was asked to write a report on the living conditions and health of the poor people in our towns and countryside.

2 There had just been a terrible epidemic of CHOLERA in 1831. Cholera is a dreadful disease. Some people thought that it had something to do with unhealthy living conditions. They asked me to investigate.

3 It took me some years to research the report. I gave it to the government in 1842. I became convinced that there was a link between filth and disease. If you read Source 9, you will see what I recommended.

4 The government didn't want to take my report seriously. It would cost too much money to put my recommendations into practice! This is where the great Dr Snow proved to be so helpful. In 1854 cholera came back and John Snow proved beyond doubt that cholera was caused by infected water. Read in Source 10 what John Snow discovered.

5 Dr Snow removed the handle of the water pump in Broad Street and no more cases of cholera occurred. He later found out how the water had become infected.

A CESSPOOL, full of raw sewage, one metre away from the pump had a cracked lining. Its contents were seeping into the drinking water.

My report had said that disease was due to the foul conditions that people lived in. John Snow's research proved it. If my portrait goes into the Hall of Fame, then it must go alongside that of Dr John Snow.

6 We are important because we made governments worry about Public Health. Just twenty years later they passed the 1875 Public Health Act, which forced all local councils to provide clean water, sewers, and to have a Medical Officer of Health.

■ DISCUSS

1 List all of the threats to health that you can see in Source 8.
2 Why was Source 8 published in the 1840s? Use Source 9 and your knowledge to explain your answer.
3 Read Source 9. What were Chadwick's *four* recommendations?
4 How did Snow help Chadwick?
5 How long did it take the government to take notice of Chadwick's recommendations?
6 Why did it take so long?

■ ACTIVITY

7 Fill out score cards for Edwin Chadwick and John Snow.

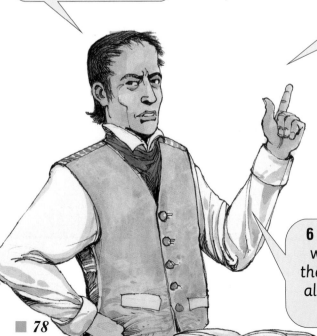

▼ **SOURCE 8** *A Court for King Cholera*, a drawing of London in the 1840s

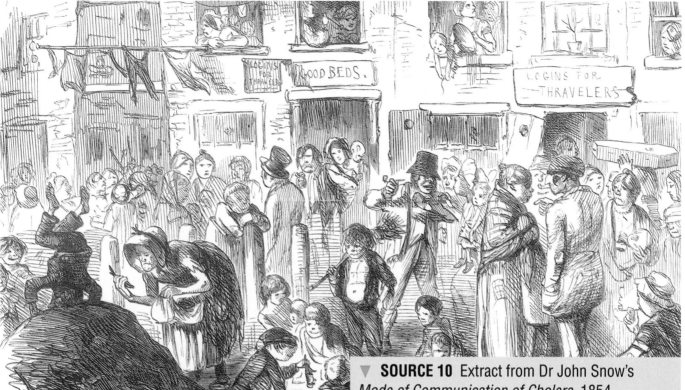

▼ **SOURCE 10** Extract from Dr John Snow's *Mode of Communication of Cholera*, 1854

The most terrible outbreak of cholera which ever occurred in this kingdom took place in Broad Street (London) a few weeks ago. There were upwards of five hundred fatal attacks of cholera in ten days. A great number of cases died within a few hours of each other.

I found that nearly all the deaths had taken place within a short distance of a particular water pump. There were only ten deaths in houses situated nearer to another street pump. In five of these cases, the family told me they always used the Broad Street Pump anyway. In the other cases it was children who went to school near the pump in Broad Street.

I conclude that the deaths from cholera are due to the evacuations [faeces and urine] finding their way from patients already infected with the disease, into the drinking water collected from the pump in Broad Street.

▼ **SOURCE 9** From Edwin Chadwick's Report

(i) Epidemic diseases are caused by decaying animal and vegetable substances, by damp and filth, and close and overcrowded dwellings. The annual loss of life from filth and bad ventilation is greater than the loss from death or wounds in any war . . .

(ii) the most important and practical steps to take are drainage, the removal of all rubbish from the streets and the improvement of the supplies of water. The expense of public drainage and supplies of water would save money because there would be less money spent on sickness and mortality [death].

(iii) to prevent further disease a district medical officer should be appointed for each area.

Medical Marvels Candidate 5: Louis Pasteur

1 My name is Louis Pasteur. I am a French scientist. I solved the greatest medical mystery of all time.

I discovered germs, or bacteria as doctors and scientists call them. After thousands of years, and hundreds of crazy ideas about the causes of disease, I can now scientifically prove that germs cause many diseases. My discovery will save the lives of millions of ordinary people.

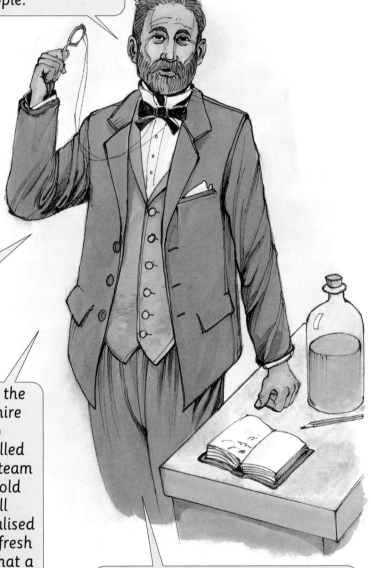

2 My research began in 1850 when I helped a brewing company to find out why their alcohol was going bad. I used a really powerful microscope to discover tiny bacteria germinating (growing) in the liquid. That is why I nicknamed these bacteria 'germs'. I tried boiling the liquid and, to my delight, these bacteria were killed. My ideas soon caught on. We discovered that these bacteria were responsible for milk, beer and vinegar going bad. So we boiled the liquids and 'pasteurised' them!

The next step was to prove that if wine and beer are changed by germs, then the same must happen sometimes in humans and animals.

3 I set up a science laboratory to continue the work of a very famous doctor whom I admire greatly – Dr Edward Jenner. I started to investigate a disease affecting chickens, called chicken cholera. One day, a member of my team accidentally injected a chicken with some old germs that had been in the laboratory all summer. When the chicken didn't die, he realised he had made a mistake. He injected it with fresh germs. It still didn't die. What a chicken! What a discovery! The old, weak germs had immunised the chicken against the disease. We had found out why Jenner's vaccines worked. Of course, I had to call this method 'vaccination', since it was Jenner's work that had put me on the right path. Some say this was just chance! I say, chance only favours the mind that is prepared!

4 I am not a doctor, I am a scientist, but my experiments and discoveries have saved the lives of millions of ordinary people. The vaccine I am most proud of protects humans from rabies.

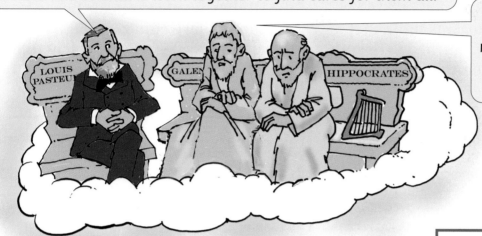

At last people will stop thinking that diseases are caused by poisonous air, the devil, bad smells, evil spirits, too much blood and other silly theories. Thanks to me, the world can look forward to a time when people understand the causes of ALL diseases and doctors and scientists work together to find cures for them all.

We were wrong! Perhaps I wasn't the most important person in the history of medicine after all.

LOUIS PASTEUR   GALEN   HIPPOCRATES

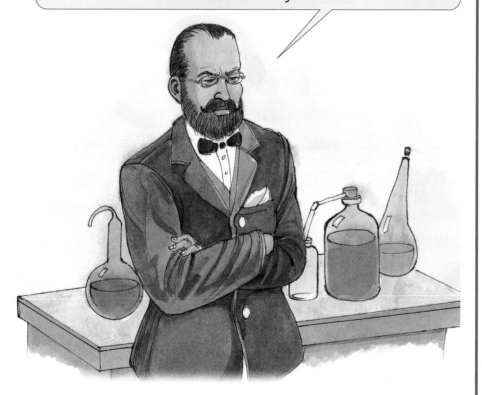

I am Robert Koch, a German scientist. If Louis Pasteur enters this Hall of Fame, then so should I. Pasteur had his theory that bacteria cause disease but who proved this theory? I did! And then I discovered vaccines to prevent cholera, tuberculosis and other diseases. Don't I deserve to be in the Hall of Fame?

■ DISCUSS

1 What was Pasteur's theory?
2 Why was this theory such an important turning point in the history of medicine?
3 Why was Robert Koch important in the history of medicine?
4 Why do you think Pasteur's theory persuaded governments to start spending a lot of money on improving public health?

■ ACTIVITY

5 Design a poster advertising chicken cholera vaccine. Remember, many farmers could not read very well in the nineteenth century. Your poster will have to explain what germs are and how the vaccine works, without using too many words!
6 Fill out a score card for Louis Pasteur.

Medical Marvels Candidate 6: Florence Nightingale

Florence Nightingale is one of the most famous women in history. Most people have heard of her work as a nurse in the Crimea, but many historians think that what she did after she returned to Britain from the Crimea was more important.

Florence Nightingale was born in 1820.

Her family was wealthy and her parents did not expect their daughter to get a job. All they wanted was for her to marry a rich man, have children and live happily ever after. However Florence had different plans. She believed that God wanted her to be a nurse.

1 Over the previous 100 years a lot of hospitals had been opened. In secret, so that her parents did not know, Florence Nightingale visited hospitals and read about them.
Conditions in many were awful.

> No one knows how to look after her. That nurse is drunk! Bringing her here is as good as giving her poison.

2 Florence Nightingale told her family that she was going to be a nurse.

> A nurse!

> You might as well be a servant!

> You can't expect me to hang about the house all my life. I will go out and work. You must look on me as if I were your son.

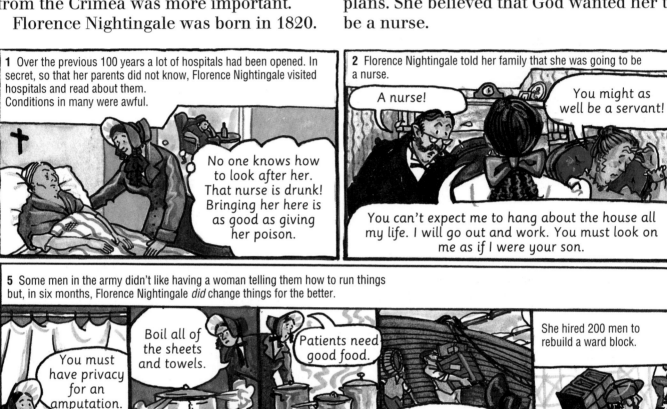

5 Some men in the army didn't like having a woman telling them how to run things but, in six months, Florence Nightingale *did* change things for the better.

> You must have privacy for an amputation.

> Boil all of the sheets and towels.

> Patients need good food.

> We need those things now! I'll pay for them myself.

She hired 200 men to rebuild a ward block.

8 But she travelled under a false name on a different ship. She avoided all the publicity. She had other plans.

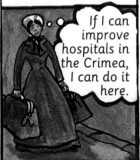

> If I can improve hospitals in the Crimea, I can do it here.

9 Florence went to see the Queen. Then she gave an 800-page report to the government, telling them about everything that had to be changed.

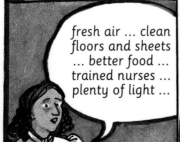

> fresh air ... clean floors and sheets ... better food ... trained nurses ... plenty of light ...

10 In three years the death rate in British army hospitals was cut by half.

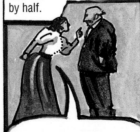

> I told you I could improve the hospitals.

11 In 1860, Florence Nightingale published her *Notes for Nursing*. It was a bestseller.

> It's very practical. This one has an extra section on looking after babies.

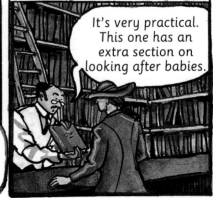

■ DISCUSS

1 What did Florence Nightingale's methods have in common with the ideas of Edwin Chadwick?
2 How did her work affect hospitals?
3 How did her work affect nurses?
4 Why do you think Pasteur's theory (pages 80–81) made it easier for Florence Nightingale to improve the conditions in hospitals?

■ ACTIVITY

5 Fill out a score card for Florence Nightingale.

---

3 In 1851, Florence secretly went to Germany to work in a hospital for three months. Then, back in London, she got her first job running a hospital for sick 'gentle-women'. It was not what she really wanted. The patients in the hospital were rich; Florence wanted to help the poor. But it was a start.

In 1854, war broke out between Russia and Britain around the Black Sea. The British army set up hospitals to care for the wounded, but conditions were so bad that almost half of the wounded soldiers brought into the army hospitals died there. Something had to be done.

A member of the British government asked Florence Nightingale for help. She agreed to lead a group of trained nurses to the Crimea.

4 The conditions in the army hospitals were even worse than Florence Nightingale had expected.

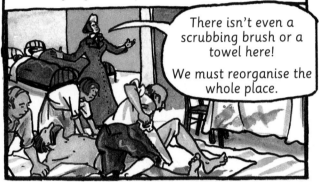

There isn't even a scrubbing brush or a towel here!

We must reorganise the whole place.

6 In six months, Florence Nightingale had cut the death rate of wounded soldiers to only two out of every hundred.

The newspapers back in Britain called her The Lady with the Lamp.

Supporters raised thousands of pounds so that she could carry on with her improvements.

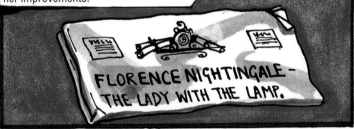

FLORENCE NIGHTINGALE – THE LADY WITH THE LAMP.

7 After two years in the Crimea, Florence returned to Britain. She was a heroine. The newspapers wanted her story . . .

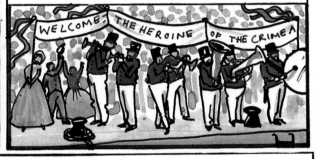

WELCOME — THE HEROINE OF THE CRIMEA

12 In the same year, Britain's first Training School for nurses was set up by Florence Nightingale with money raised for her while she was in the Crimea.

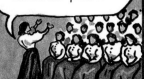

I'll show you how to make ordinary hospitals into better, healthier places.

13 Whenever a new hospital was being built its designers would ask advice from Florence. She showed them how to lay out a hospital so that nurses could do their job better.

She even improved conditions in workhouse hospitals.

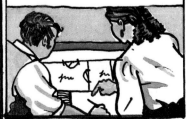

14 In 1907 her lifetime's work was recognised – she was given the Order of Merit. She died, aged ninety, in 1910.

In Victorian times, women were expected to stay in the background and let men make all the decisions. Florence Nightingale refused to do this and, as a result, hospitals in Britain became much healthier places.

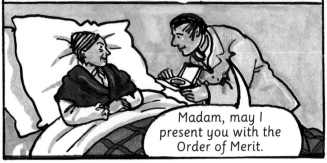

Madam, may I present you with the Order of Merit.

Medical Marvels Candidate 7: Joseph Lister

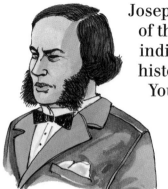

Joseph Lister was one of the most important individuals in the history of surgery. You might even owe your life to him!

■ **DISCUSS**

1 How did Lister's background help him?
2 What was Lister's great discovery?
3 How was his work helped by the discoveries of Pasteur and Koch?

■ **ACTIVITY 1**

4 Fill out a score card for Joseph Lister.

What was Lister's background?

- His father developed better microscopes.
- Lister had the best medical training. He learned to challenge existing ideas. He did research into infected wounds.
- He became a surgeon in Glasgow and later in London.

What did Lister discover?

- Even after successful operations, patients often died because their wounds became infected. Lister solved this problem.
- In 1867 Lister read Pasteur's work on bacteria. He thought that bacteria might be causing the infections. He used CARBOLIC SPRAY to kill these bacteria. This was antiseptic surgery.

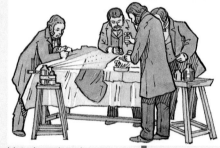

Lister's antiseptic surgery

Why was Lister's work important?

In the short term

- More of his patients survived. The percentage of his patients who died after operations fell from 46 per cent to 15 per cent.

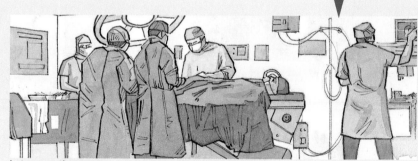

Later: aseptic surgery

- His ideas spread and were used by other doctors, although at first many doctors did not believe in Lister's discovery.

In the long term

- Other doctors built on his ideas. Hospitals and operating theatres became much cleaner places. All medical instruments were sterilised effectively. The whole room was sterile. All germs were killed. This was called ASEPTIC surgery.
- Longer and more complicated operations became possible as the danger of infection was reduced.

Before you make your choices for the Medical Marvels Hall of Fame . . .

So who does deserve to be in the Medical Marvels of the Millennium Hall of Fame? You may have already decided who was the most important, but now think about the links between them. The diagram below shows some questions you need to think about and discuss before making up your mind and choosing the four people whose portraits will go up on the walls of your Hall of Fame (see pages 70–71).

(see pages 70–71)

■ **ACTIVITY 2**

5 Make your own copy of this diagram. Add arrows and labels to show the links between the 'marvels'. You can use the questions below, but you might be able to add other links of your own, too.

Joseph Lister — Edward Jenner — Florence Nightingale — James Simpson — Louis Pasteur — Edwin Chadwick

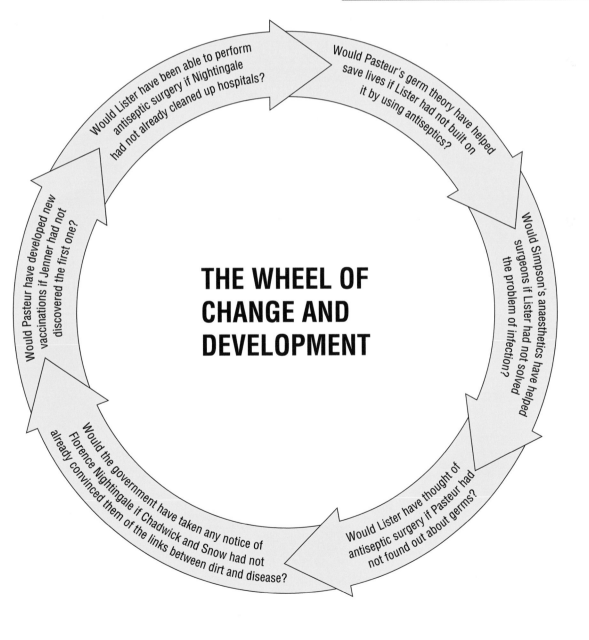

THE WHEEL OF CHANGE AND DEVELOPMENT

Would Lister have been able to perform antiseptic surgery if Nightingale had not already cleaned up hospitals?

Would Pasteur's germ theory have helped save lives if Lister had not built on it by using antiseptics?

Would Simpson's anaesthetics have helped surgeons if Lister had not solved the problem of infection?

Would Lister have thought of antiseptic surgery if Pasteur had not found out about germs?

Would the government have taken any notice of Florence Nightingale if Chadwick and Snow had not already convinced them of the links between dirt and disease?

Would Pasteur have developed new vaccinations if Jenner had not discovered the first one?

4.3 *What factors made the medical revolution possible?*

The discoveries that you have been reading about on pages 72–85 did not happen by accident. There were several factors that helped them to take place. Can you work out what they were?

1 Doctors' attitudes changed. Once they realised that the old idea about the four humours was wrong they began to look for different explanations for diseases.

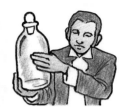

2 Florence Nightingale was motivated to make people healthier because of her religious beliefs.

3 Louis Pasteur was a scientist. He developed his ideas whilst working for the brewing industry. He used all the latest technology to do his research. It was only afterwards that he applied his scientific discoveries to human diseases.

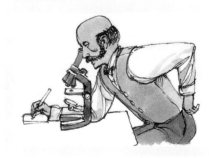

■ ACTIVITY

1 On these pages are nine boxes. Each one is telling you about a factor that helped to change medicine. But which factor? Copy and complete the table below, identifying at least one factor for each box. These are the factors you are looking for.

The factors
- Attitudes and religious beliefs
- War
- Governments
- Communications
- Science and technology
- Individual genius

Box	Factors	How it helped lead to these discoveries (look back at pages 72–85 for examples)
1		

■ DISCUSS

2 Which of the developments in the boxes are linked back to developments that began during the Medical Renaissance? Explain how they are linked.

3 Which TWO factors do you think were most important in changing medicine between 1750 and 1900?

4 Improvements in glass-making technology led to better microscopes which helped Pasteur discover germs. Developments in steel-making helped to produce a thin syringe needle that did not break, which could be used for vaccinations.

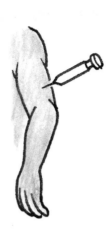

5 Government got more involved in public health. Politicians realised that they had to make laws to force people to become more healthy – laws such as compulsory vaccinations and making all towns build sewers. One hundred years before, politicians would never have dreamed of interfering like this.

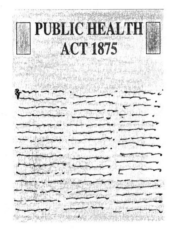

6 There was a revolution in communications in the nineteenth century. Details of Pasteur's experiments were quickly reported in newspapers. Fast boat and train travel allowed doctors to meet at national conferences and learn from each others' ideas.

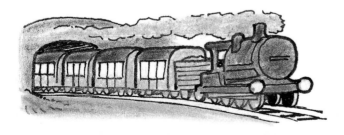

7 Florence Nightingale learned her skills because she was sent to help soldiers fighting in the Crimean War. She persuaded the government to clean up hospitals because they needed healthy soldiers to fight in wars.

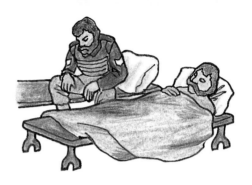

8 Jenner, Simpson and Lister were all talented doctors. Chadwick and Nightingale were talented and forceful campaigners. Pasteur was a scientific genius. They were all ambitious individuals who worked hard to make changes and get their ideas accepted.

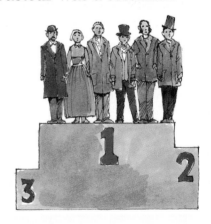

9 The French government gave lots of money to Pasteur to do his research because they wanted him to do better than their enemies the Germans.

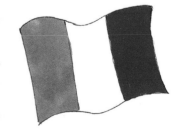

CHAPTER 5   *Medicine since 1900*

▼ **SOURCE 1** Improvements in life expectancy in the UK, 1900–2000

Average age at death

1900

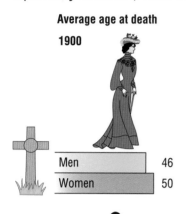

Men	46
Women	50

1930

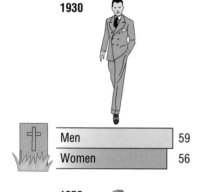

Men	59
Women	56

1950

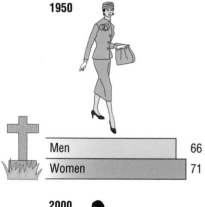

Men	66
Women	71

2000

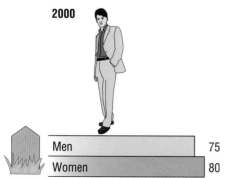

Men	75
Women	80

Despite all of the discoveries and improvements in medicine during the nineteenth century there were still big problems to solve. As you can see from the timeline in Source 1, life expectancy in 1900 was still much lower than it is today. Many people, especially the poor, could not expect to live beyond 50. In the twentieth century life expectancy in the UK increased to 75. This chapter will help you to work out why.

1 What have been the major improvements in medicine and health since 1900 and how have they helped?
2 Why have these improvements happened?

Page 89 gives you an idea of these improvements.

■ ACTIVITY

Complete your own copy of the table below.

1 Write out the problems **in your own words** in Column A.
2 Fill in Column B by choosing the solution from the solution box that fits each problem.
3 Now think about Column C. Which factors do you think helped to produce each solution? These are your first ideas. Through the chapter you can find out if you were right, and add any more ideas to your table.

Column A – Problems	Column B – Solutions	Column C – Factors
1 Infant deaths –		
2 Cost of treatment –		
3 Housing –		
4 Infections –		
5 Bleeding –		

■ DISCUSS

4 Which factor do you expect to be most important in improving medicine and increasing life expectancy between 1900 and 2000?

The problems in 1900

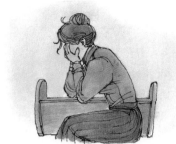

1 In 1900, 163 out of every 1000 babies (around 16 per cent) died before their first birthday.

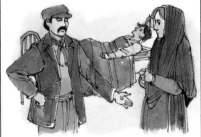

2 People had to pay to go to a doctor and most families could not afford the cost.

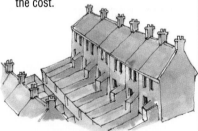

3 Many families still lived in unhealthy houses.

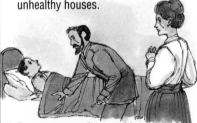

4 Doctors were often unable to cure patients because there was no way of fighting infections inside the body.

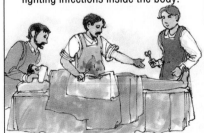

5 Doctors had not solved the problems caused by high blood loss during an operation or after an accident.

The solutions

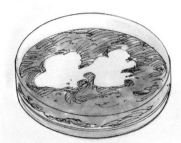

A Antibiotics such as penicillin were discovered and developed.

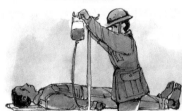

B Scientists and doctors discovered that people had different BLOOD GROUPS, which meant that BLOOD TRANSFUSIONS could now take place successfully.

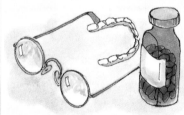

C The NATIONAL HEALTH SERVICE was set up in 1948, giving everyone free medical advice and treatment.

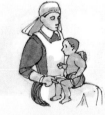

D Mothers and children had cleaner houses, better food, medical care from trained MIDWIVES and vaccination against disease.

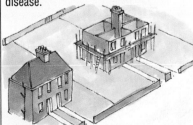

E Slums were cleared and new, better houses were built.

The factors

Attitudes and religious beliefs

War

Governments

Communications

Science and technology

Individual genius

5.1 *How have wars affected medicine since 1900?*

There were two world wars in the twentieth century. They caused great suffering and millions of people died. However, they also led to medical progress. Pages 90–93 explain how this happened and help you to write an essay summarising the links between war and medical progress.

■ **DISCUSS**

1 List all the medical problems you can see in Source 1.
2 What questions do you need to ask about Source 1 before deciding whether it is useful evidence for a historian?
3 Do you think the painting contains useful evidence about medical problems in the First World War? Explain the reasons for your answer.

The First World War

During the First World War more people were killed and wounded than in any previous war. New and deadly weapons were used for the first time, such as SHRAPNEL bombs and high-explosive shells. They caused terrible injuries that surgeons had never seen before.

▼ **SOURCE 1** *The Harvest of Battle*. This painting shows wounded soldiers making their way across a battlefield to a hospital tent. It was painted in 1919 by C. R. W. Nevinson. Nevinson joined the Belgian Red Cross in 1914 and worked as a stretcher-bearer in France. He later became an official war artist

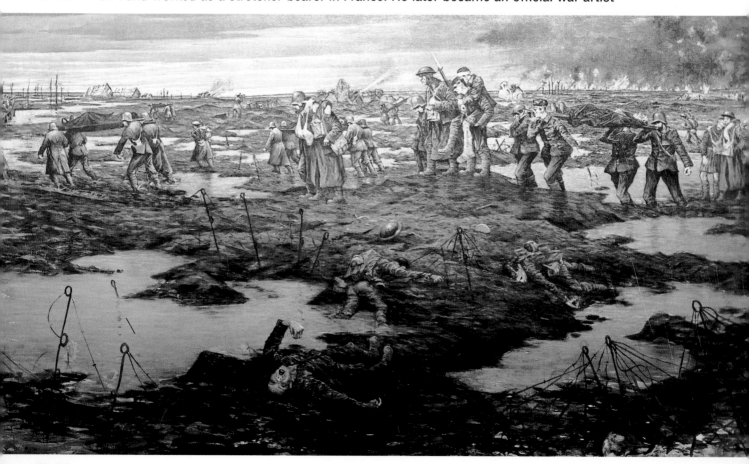

■ ACTIVITY

4 Look at Source 2. Find one discovery made before the war that was developed more quickly because of the war. Explain why war speeded up its development.

5 Copy the table below. Complete the middle column using Source 2 to help you.

6 Fill in the third column. You don't need to fill in every row but you should be able to find examples of how the following factors helped to improve medicine.

- ■ Attitudes and religious beliefs
- ■ Governments
- ■ Communications
- ■ Science and technology

Problem	How did medicine improve as a result?	Which other factors played a part in this improvement?
Head wounds and brain damage were very common		
Bullets and shrapnel got lodged deep in soldiers' wounds		
Soldiers bled to death while waiting for an operation		
Many recruits were very unhealthy		

▼ **SOURCE 2** How the First World War improved medicine and health

Millions were wounded, giving surgeons the opportunity to experiment with new techniques.

Surgeons developed new techniques to repair broken bones, and to perform SKIN GRAFTS – which formed the basis for PLASTIC SURGERY.

Head wounds were particularly common. Surgery of the eye, ear, nose and throat all improved rapidly. Brain surgery advanced.

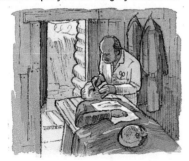

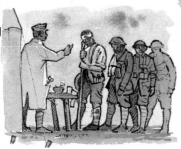

Many of the surgeons who learned their skills quickly in wartime worked as specialist surgeons after the war.

X-RAYS were discovered before the war. During the war they were used very successfully to find bullets and shrapnel lodged in the body. Governments paid for more and more X-ray machines to be made.

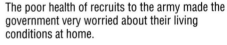

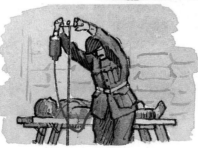

The deep wounds made by bombs and machine-gun fire meant that many soldiers were bleeding to death before they could be operated on. Blood transfusion was used effectively for the first time. Methods of storing blood and transporting it were improved.

The poor health of recruits to the army made the government very worried about their living conditions at home.

The soldiers who fought in the war were promised 'homes fit for heroes' when they returned. This speeded up the process of getting rid of unhealthy slum housing in Britain.

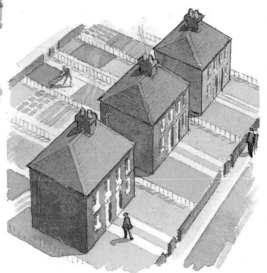

The Second World War

Civilians were far more likely to be killed or injured in the Second World War than the First World War because of the increased threat of bombs. However, in spite of these casualties, the Second World War also helped medicine to advance because doctors, surgeons and governments had to find ways of:

1 saving soldiers whose wounds had become infected
2 helping civilians. This meant that public health services had to be dramatically improved.

Here are some of the effects of the Second World War on medicine and health:

■ **DISCUSS**

Look at the effects of the Second World War on medicine and health shown below.

1 Which improvements helped soldiers most?
2 Which improvements helped civilians most?
3 Which factor apart from war played the biggest part in these improvements?

Blood transfusion
There were more improvements. Blood could be stored for longer. Civilians donated blood.

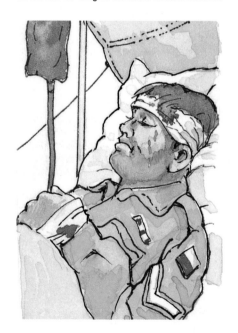

Diet
RATIONING was introduced to improve some people's diet. Government posters encouraged healthy eating.

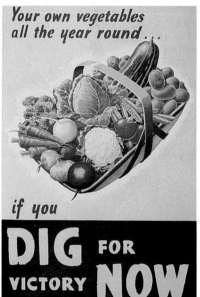

Your own vegetables all the year round ...

if you **DIG** FOR **NOW** VICTORY

Drugs
Penicillin was developed – the first antibiotic.

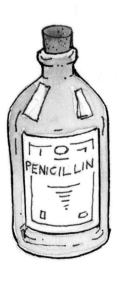

▼ **SOURCE 3** The views of Heneage Ogilvey, a British surgeon

In wartime, industry spends more time and money on developing new surgical equipment

Surgeons do more operations and are prepared to work harder in wartime than in peacetime

WHY DOES **WAR** IMPROVE **SURGERY**?

In peacetime surgeons sometimes work alone and in competition against each other. In war they unite and share ideas to help their own soldiers

■ **ACTIVITY**

4 Using the information you have collected about both world wars, write an essay entitled:

How has war helped medicine to improve since 1900?

Use these questions to help you to write five paragraphs for your essay:

Paragraph 1 Which of the problems listed in column 1 on page 89 did war help to solve? (Look at page 89 for some clues.)

Paragraph 2 How did war help to improve surgery? (Source 3 will help with this.)

Paragraph 3 How did war help to make better use of inventions and discoveries? (Look at page 91.)

Paragraph 4 How did war help to improve civilian health? (Pages 91, 92 and 93 will help.)

Paragraph 5 Which other factors combined with war to help to make improvements? (Look back to the Activity on page 91 and Question 3 of the Discuss box on page 92 to help with this paragraph.)

Poverty
To be safe, 1.5 million children were moved from their homes in the cities into rural areas. This showed all too clearly the huge contrast between the living standards of rich and poor. It made the government even more determined to fight poverty more seriously after the war.

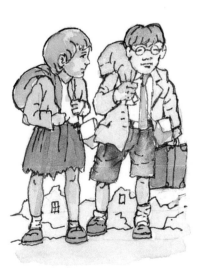

Surgery
Surgeons made advances in the use of skin grafts (which led to plastic surgery) and in the treatment of burns.

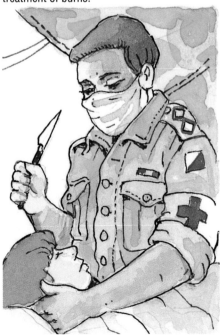

The National Health Service
The government made lots of improvements to health services for civilians. In 1942 William Beveridge, a leading civil servant, put forward the idea that these should be continued after the war as a 'free national health service' for everyone.

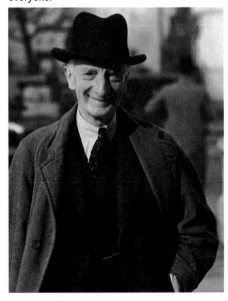

5.2 *How have governments affected medicine since 1900?*

Since the middle of the nineteenth century, governments in Britain have become more involved in improving people's health. In this enquiry you are going to discover how they helped in the twentieth century and how other factors also contributed.

▼ **SOURCE 1** How the National Insurance scheme worked

The 1911 National Insurance Act said that workers, employers and the government must all pay money into a sickness fund.

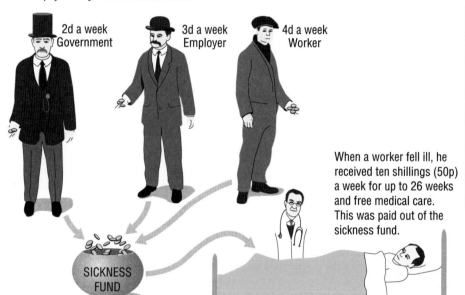

2d a week
Government

3d a week
Employer

4d a week
Worker

SICKNESS FUND

When a worker fell ill, he received ten shillings (50p) a week for up to 26 weeks and free medical care. This was paid out of the sickness fund.

■ **DISCUSS**

1 **a)** What did the National Insurance Act do?
  b) Why was it an important step forward?
2 What does Source 2 tell you about the success of National Insurance?
3 Why did governments' attitudes to housing change?
4 How did war help to pave the way for the National Health Service?
5 What was so different about the NHS from medical services before 1948?

Improvement 1: National Insurance

At the beginning of the twentieth century the poor and unemployed could not afford to get help if they were sick. The first step towards helping them came in 1911 when the Liberal government passed the National Insurance Act. The aim was to give workers the chance to get medical help and sick pay if they could not work because they were ill. Source 1 shows how the scheme worked. It was a start, but it was very limited. It only applied to people in work. The unemployed, long-term sick and the elderly could not pay into the scheme, so they could not get help. People like Kathleen Davys (Source 2) still could not afford a doctor.

▼ **SOURCE 2** From an interview in the 1930s with Kathleen Davys, one of a family of thirteen children. She lived in Birmingham. The local doctor charged sixpence (2½p) per visit

For headaches, we had vinegar and brown paper. For whooping cough we had camphorated oil rubbed on our chests or goose fat. For mumps we had stockings round our throats and measles we had tea stewed in the teapot by the fire – all different kinds of home cures. They thought they were better than going to the doctor's. Well, they couldn't afford the doctor because sixpence in those days was like looking at a five pound note today.

Improvement 2: Better Housing

In 1900 poor housing was still a major cause of ill health. Many houses did not have fresh water piped in and did not have toilets. In the early 1900s governments started to improve building standards but the first big step forward came with the Housing Act in 1919. This came after the First World War, when the government had promised to provide 'homes fit for heroes' as the soldiers came home. The Housing Act said that local councils had to provide good homes for working people to rent. A quarter of a million new houses were built under this scheme. The next step was to clear the overcrowded, filthy slums where there were the biggest problems of disease and poor health. This began in the 1930s. Tens of thousands of slum houses were cleared and 700,000 new homes were built. Even so, the last of the slums did not disappear until the 1960s.

Improvement 3: National Health Service

The Second World War, in which people of all classes worked closely together, led to a call for a fairer, better health service that would help everyone, not just those who could afford to pay to see a doctor.

As a result a leading civil servant, William Beveridge, put forward a plan in 1942 to reform medical services. After the war, Beveridge's plan led to the creation of the National Health Service in 1948. The key point was that all services were free. Doctors, dentists and nurses were to be paid by the government instead of by their patients. Hospitals would be paid for by the government, not by charity collections and local taxes. This was the biggest step forward in improving the health of people in Britain.

▼ **SOURCE 3** Services provided by the National Health Service

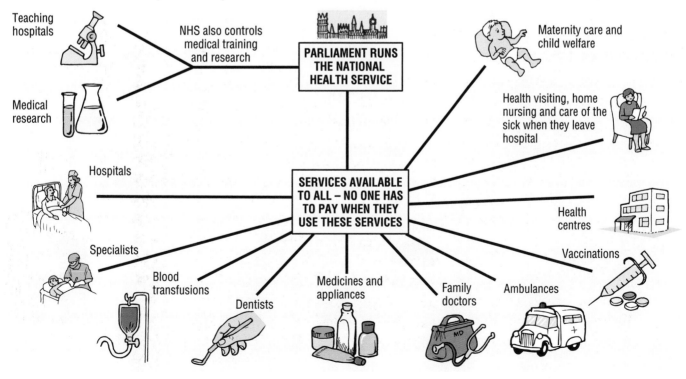

5.3 *Why did infant mortality fall so rapidly after 1900?*

One of the most dramatic improvements of the twentieth century was the reduction in the number of babies who died before they reached their first birthday. Find out why.

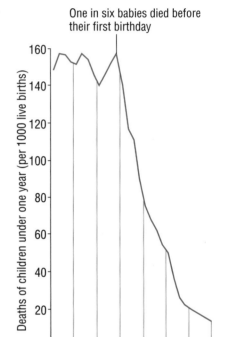

One in six babies died before their first birthday

Deaths of children under one year (per 1000 live births)

Year

■ **ACTIVITY**

1 Complete your own copy of this table:

Problems	Solutions

a) In the first column write down the problems (see below).
b) Match each problem to one or more solutions given opposite and write the solutions in the second column. Some problems have more than one solution.
2 Which of the following factors played a part in cutting infant mortality? Explain your choices.

- Attitudes and beliefs
- War
- Governments
- Communications
- Science and technology
- Individual genius

Problems leading to high levels of infant mortality

Housing

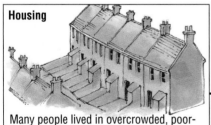

Many people lived in overcrowded, poor-quality housing. These houses were damp, dirty and had no toilets.

Diet

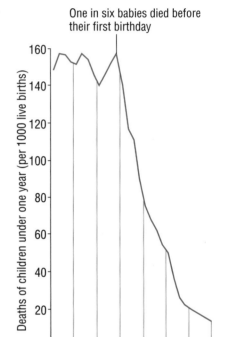

Parents and babies had poor diets.

Why was infant mortality so high?

Disease

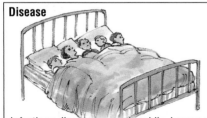

Infectious diseases spread rapidly, because vaccines had not been developed for some of the most common killer diseases.

Medical care

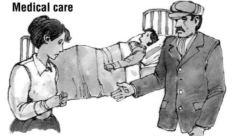

Many parents could not afford medical care.

Education

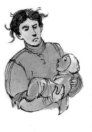

There were not enough trained midwives to help and advise new mothers. Some parents did not know how to keep their babies healthy.

Solutions to the problems leading to high infant mortality

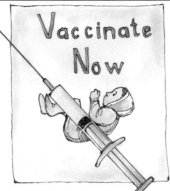

Scientists developed **new vaccines**. Governments ran national campaigns to make sure that all children were vaccinated. For example, compulsory vaccination against diphtheria in 1940 reduced deaths from 300 per million to less than 10 per million.

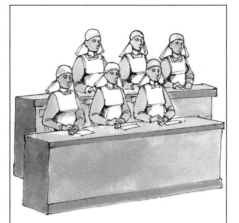

In 1902 the government said that all **midwives** had to be trained.

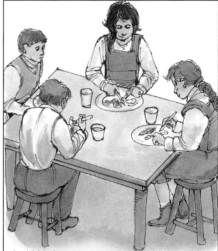

In 1906 the government started to provide **school meals**, so that children of poor families could get some good food.

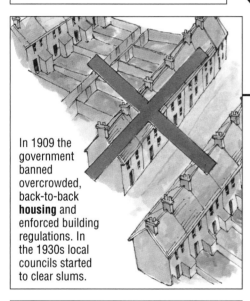

In 1909 the government banned overcrowded, back-to-back **housing** and enforced building regulations. In the 1930s local councils started to clear slums.

Why has infant mortality fallen?

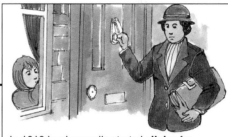

In 1919 local councils started **clinics** for mothers to be. They appointed **health visitors** to visit families and advise on health and hygiene.

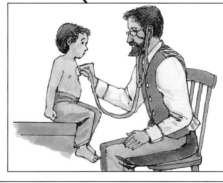

In 1944 the development of penicillin began the story of **antibiotics**. Since then antibiotics have protected babies and young children against infections that might have killed them in 1900.

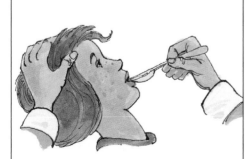

In 1948 the **National Health Service** was set up. It provided free medical treatment and medicines for everyone.

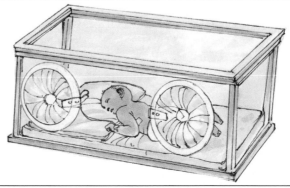

Since the 1970s **technology** has advanced greatly: babies can now be scanned before they are born to check that they are healthy and premature babies can be kept alive when they would have died in 1900.

5.4 *How was penicillin developed?*

So far in this chapter you have been looking at broad themes within medicine. Now you are going to look at a single event – one of the greatest breakthroughs in medical history – the development of penicillin. At page 101 you will draw a chart showing how different factors linked together to make this possible.

■ ACTIVITY

Read the story of penicillin on pages 98–100. Make a list of the factors that played a part in its discovery and development.

What is penicillin?

Penicillin is a drug that cures infections. This type of drug is called an antibiotic. It is used to kill bacteria. We now have hundreds of antibiotics, but penicillin was the first.

When was penicillin discovered?

Penicillin was first discovered during the nineteenth century but no one knew how useful it could be. Then in 1928 a scientist, Alexander Fleming, made a very important discovery …

▼ **SOURCE 1** A. Maurois, *The Life of Sir Alexander Fleming*, 1963

Fleming was in his little laboratory as usual, surrounded by countless dishes [the containers used by scientists to grow bacteria in]. Fleming took several old dishes and removed the lids. Several had been contaminated with mould … 'As soon as you uncover a CULTURE dish,' said Fleming, 'something tiresome is sure to happen. Things fall out of the air.' Suddenly he stopped talking, then, after a moment said … 'That's funny …' On one of the cultures there was a growth of mould, as on several others, but on this particular one, all around the mould the colonies of bacteria had been dissolved …

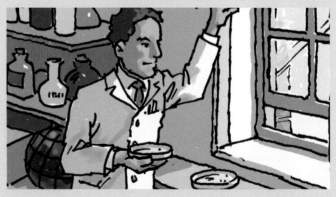

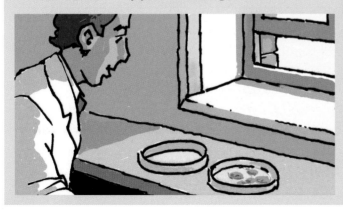

The penicillin bacteria had, by some miraculous chance, blown in through an open window. It had then killed the other bacteria being grown in the dish!

How was penicillin developed?

Unfortunately Fleming did not have enough money or government support to continue experimenting with penicillin. So nothing was done about his chance discovery for another ten years. It was the Second World War that finally persuaded the government to fund further experiments with penicillin. Three days after the war began, two scientists from Oxford University, Howard Florey and Ernst Chain, got some government money to research into penicillin. They had read Fleming's article and devised a method to make and test penicillin.

Stage 1: growing the penicillin

Thousands of milk bottles were used to grow the penicillin bacteria. This produced a few grams of pure penicillin that were collected using a hand pump.

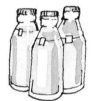

Stage 2: testing the penicillin on animals

Eight mice were injected with dangerous germs. Four mice were then given penicillin. Four were not. The next day the mice who had been injected with penicillin were fine. The others were dead.

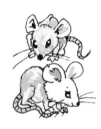

Stage 3: the first human trial of penicillin

The team had to go back to the milk bottles and grow some more penicillin. This took a long time. It wasn't until February 1941 that there was enough to test on a human patient. Source 2 tells you about that test.

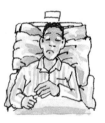

▼ **SOURCE 2** Professor Fletcher (one of Florey's team) remembering the events of 1941

The patient had a sore on his mouth a month previously, and the infection had spread to his scalp. He'd had an ABSCESS there. It had spread to both his eyes and one had to be removed. He had abscesses open on his arm. He had an abscess on his lung – he was well on his way towards death from a terrible infection. We'd nothing to lose and everything to gain. So we thought we'd try penicillin.

There was so little penicillin that after the first day I collected his urine and I took it over to where Florey was working so that the penicillin could be taken from the urine and used again.

On the fourth day the patient was really dramatically improved, he was sitting up in bed and his temperature had gone down. On the fifth day the penicillin began to run out and we couldn't go on. Of course when they took it from the urine they couldn't get it all back and it gradually ran out . . . He eventually died.

How was penicillin mass-produced?

Although the patient died, the trial showed just how powerful penicillin could be if the scientists could find a way of growing huge amounts. By December 1941, the Americans had joined the Second World War. The next year, the American government gave $80 million to four drug companies to find a way to mass-produce penicillin. Two years later they had made the first batches.

In 1943 the scientists used penicillin to treat wounded British soldiers for the first time.

> ▼ **SOURCE 3** Lt Colonel Pulvertaft describes the first use of penicillin by the British Army in 1943
>
> *The first man I tried it on was called Newton. He had been in bed for six months with compound fractures of both legs. His sheets were soaked with pus and heat made the smell intolerable. Normally he would have died in a short time. I gave three injections a day of penicillin and studied the effects under a microscope ... the thing seemed like a miracle. In ten days' time the leg was cured.*

By June 1944 there was enough penicillin to treat all the casualties from D-Day, when the Allied armies invaded France.

If they had not been given penicillin many more soldiers would have died from infected wounds. By 1945, the American army was using two million doses a month. It is estimated that penicillin saved 12–15 per cent of soldiers' lives during the Second World War.

As soon as the war was over, penicillin became available for civilian use. Nowadays, most people have taken penicillin or similar antibiotic drugs at some point in their lives. It is used to cure meningitis, pneumonia, chest infections, throat infections, abscesses, kidney infections, cuts and infections caught after operations. Penicillin really can be called the wonder drug of the twentieth century.

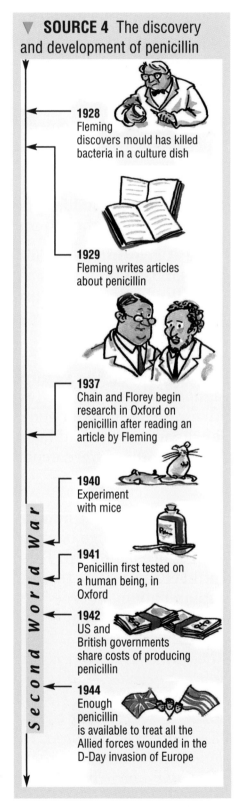

▼ **SOURCE 4** The discovery and development of penicillin

1928
Fleming discovers mould has killed bacteria in a culture dish

1929
Fleming writes articles about penicillin

1937
Chain and Florey begin research in Oxford on penicillin after reading an article by Fleming

1940
Experiment with mice

1941
Penicillin first tested on a human being, in Oxford

1942
US and British governments share costs of producing penicillin

1944
Enough penicillin is available to treat all the Allied forces wounded in the D-Day invasion of Europe

Second World War

■ ACTIVITY

1 Copy the chart. In each box write one or two sentences explaining how the factor helped the development of penicillin.

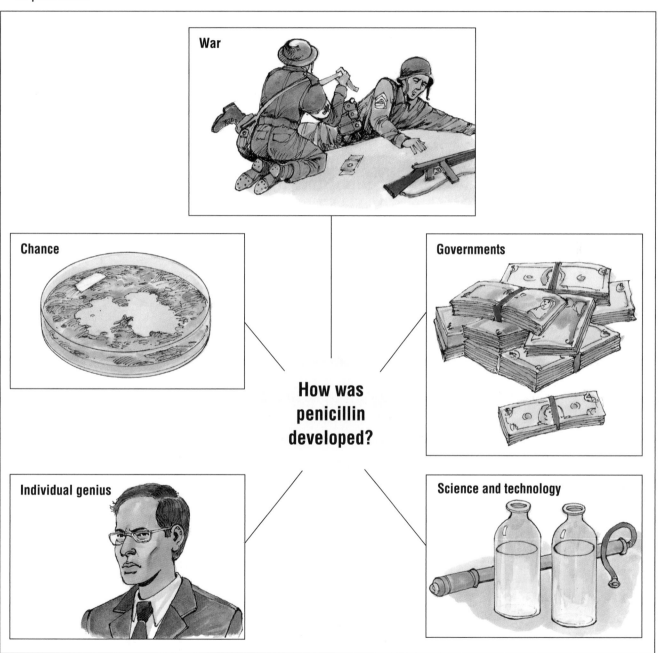

2 Can you work out any connections between the factors? Choose two factors and explain how they worked together to help to develop penicillin.

3 Which factor do you think was most important? Explain your reasons. For example, you could think about how a factor started the story of penicillin or helped to make it widely used.

5.5   *DNA – the greatest discovery of all?*

In the time you have been working through this book there will have been important medical developments. One of the most important at the moment is GENETIC ENGINEERING. It is based on the discovery of DNA and this may be the greatest discovery in the history of medicine, greater even than Pasteur's germ theory. This is your chance to find out why this breakthrough is so important.

The discovery of DNA

DNA is inside every CELL of your body. It is the code inside your GENES. Genes decide everything about you.

Even in the 1800s scientists knew that DNA existed and that it somehow controlled what we are like but that was all they knew. Then:

Stage 1: In 1953 two scientists called Francis Crick and James Watson discovered the structure of DNA and how it passed on information from parents to children.

Stage 2: In the 1990s the Human Genome Project began working out the exact contents of the DNA in the human body – finding out exactly what each part of the DNA does. The information contained in one person would fill 160,000 books like this! That's why it took ten years for scientists – working as a huge team across eighteen countries and using the latest computers – to finish the project.

What is DNA?

- Inside every cell of your body are several identical strings of DNA.
- A tiny part of your DNA looks like this:

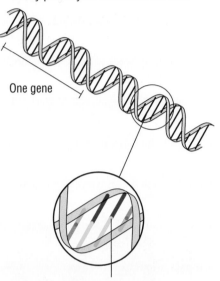

One gene

The structure of DNA is a double helix – a pair of interlocking spirals. They are joined by 'bases', set in pairs, which are like the rungs of a ladder.

- You can think of DNA as a long list of instructions like a computer program that operate every cell of your body. There are more than 3000 million letters of code in your body's program.
- These instructions are grouped together into sets of instructions called genes.
- Each gene has a different function. For example – some decide your eye colour or how much hair you have. Some decide whether you will develop a disease or disability.
- Everybody's DNA carries slightly different instructions – which is why human beings are all different.

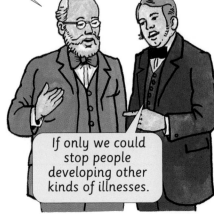

Thanks to Pasteur we know that bacteria cause disease. Now we can develop vaccines to stop people catching these infectious diseases.

If only we could stop people developing other kinds of illnesses.

1900

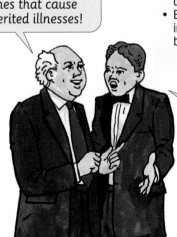

Now we understand DNA we can deal with genes that cause inherited illnesses!

But how long will it take? And which illnesses? Is it really that simple?

2000

■ ACTIVITY

1 Draw a diagram with four boxes like the one below.

2 Read the information in the diagram and decide on a suitable 'factor' heading for each box. Three of the headings should be factors you have used before in this book. One heading is a new factor.

3 Write your own sentence in each box summarising how each factor contributed to the discovery of DNA.

4 All four factors worked together to help to make the discovery of DNA. Explain in your own words how they were all connected to each other.

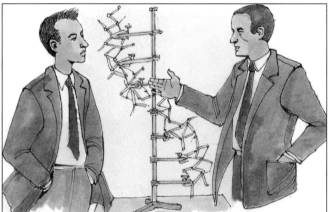

Francis Crick and James Watson were great scientists. They were both experts and were very good at working together but were also very adventurous in their ideas. They were prepared to try out ideas and methods other scientists would not try.

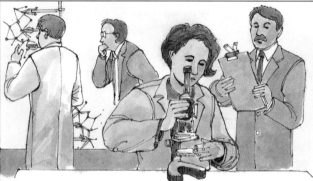

Although Crick and Watson were vital to the discovery, they did not work alone. They also had help from a team of scientists including Rosalind Franklin. This increased the skills and knowledge that helped to make the breakthrough. In the twentieth century teamwork by scientists was more important in making discoveries than scientists working alone.

> **Why was the structure of DNA discovered in 1953?**

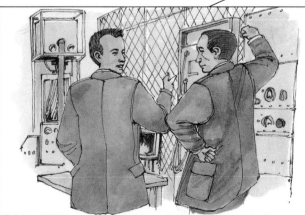

Crick and Watson were able to use the best equipment – improved microscopes, X-ray photography – and the latest knowledge in sciences such as biochemistry. Therefore they were building on all the discoveries that had taken place before.

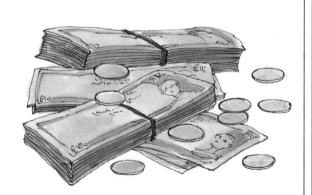

Huge sums of money were needed to pay for all the scientific work. Expensive equipment was needed and all the people involved had to be paid. Most of the money came from the government but industries also made a contribution.

6.1 *How has understanding of the causes of disease changed?*

For centuries healers have struggled to understand why people become ill. These pages summarise the different explanations for illness and disease that healers have had through history.

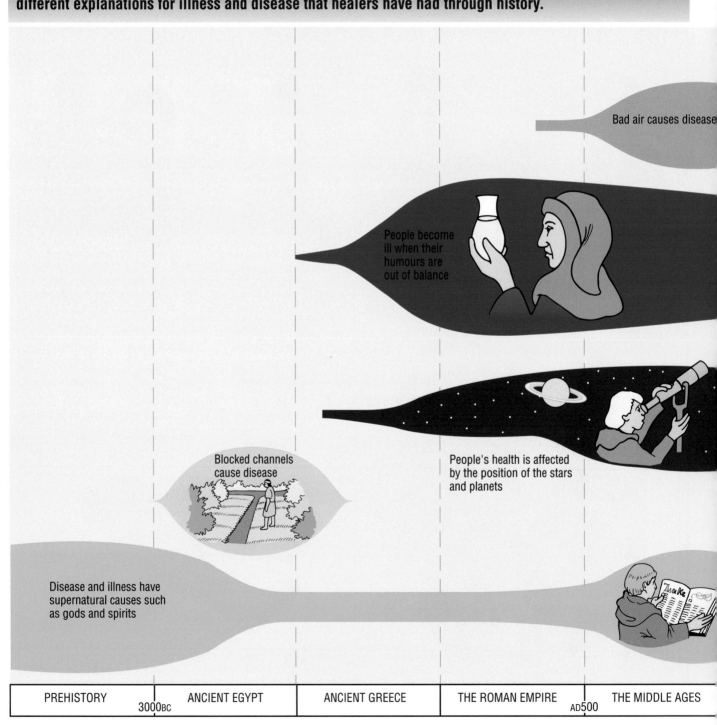

Bad air causes disease

People become ill when their humours are out of balance

People's health is affected by the position of the stars and planets

Blocked channels cause disease

Disease and illness have supernatural causes such as gods and spirits

PREHISTORY	ANCIENT EGYPT	ANCIENT GREECE	THE ROMAN EMPIRE	THE MIDDLE AGES
	3000BC		AD500	

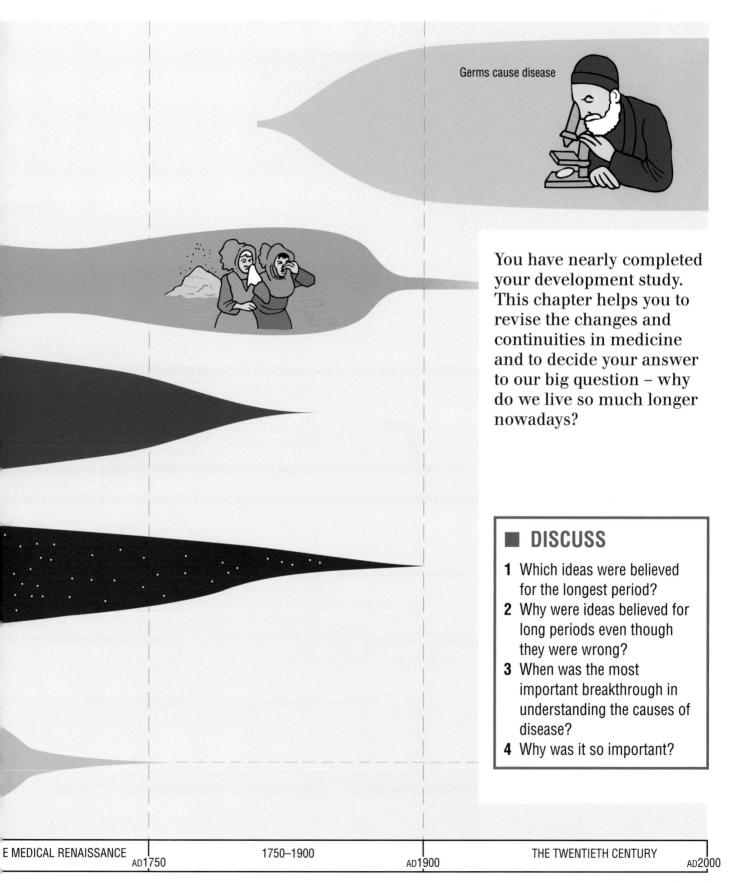

Germs cause disease

You have nearly completed your development study. This chapter helps you to revise the changes and continuities in medicine and to decide your answer to our big question – why do we live so much longer nowadays?

■ DISCUSS

1 Which ideas were believed for the longest period?

2 Why were ideas believed for long periods even though they were wrong?

3 When was the most important breakthrough in understanding the causes of disease?

4 Why was it so important?

E MEDICAL RENAISSANCE   AD1750   1750–1900   AD1900   THE TWENTIETH CENTURY   AD2000

6.2 How have methods of treatment changed?

These two pages summarise some of the main treatments that have been used across the centuries.

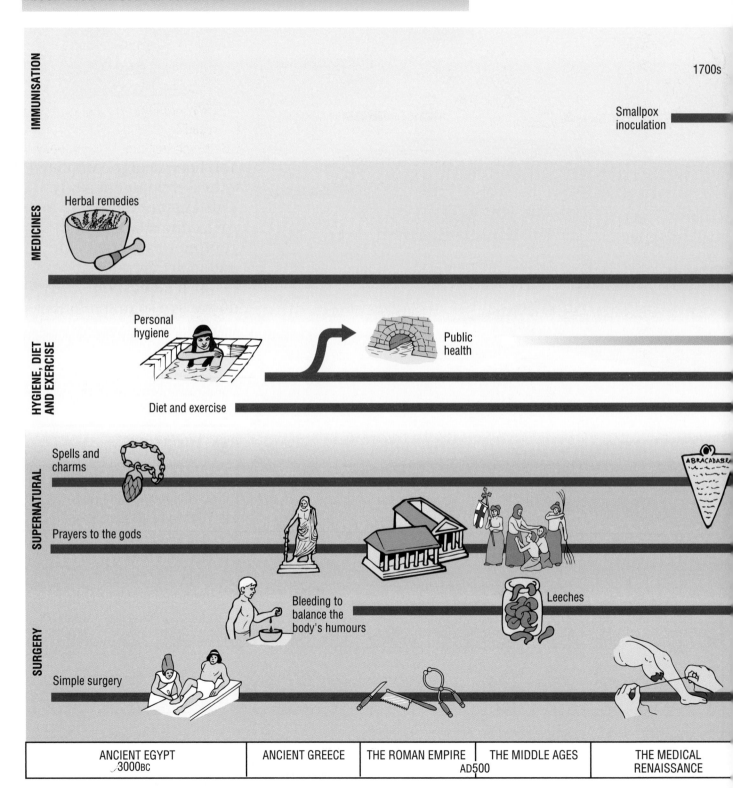

IMMUNISATION

1700s

Smallpox inoculation

MEDICINES

Herbal remedies

HYGIENE, DIET AND EXERCISE

Personal hygiene

Public health

Diet and exercise

SUPERNATURAL

Spells and charms

ABRACADABRA

Prayers to the gods

SURGERY

Bleeding to balance the body's humours

Leeches

Simple surgery

ANCIENT EGYPT 3000BC	ANCIENT GREECE	THE ROMAN EMPIRE AD500	THE MIDDLE AGES	THE MEDICAL RENAISSANCE

■ DISCUSS

1 Which treatments have been used for the greatest length of time?
2 Why have they been used for so long?
3 Which treatments used in earlier times are not used today?
4 Why are they no longer used?
5 Which treatments used today were not used in earlier times?
6 Why were they not used in earlier times?
7 When was the period of greatest change in treatments?

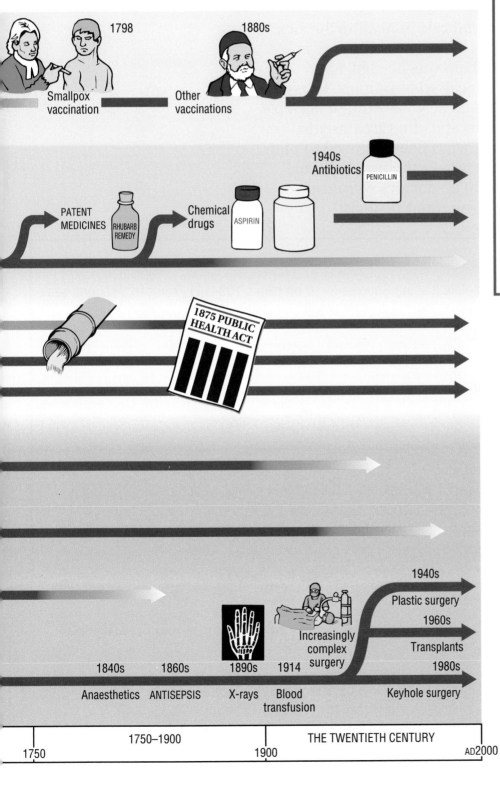

1798 Smallpox vaccination

1880s Other vaccinations

PATENT MEDICINES — RHUBARB REMEDY

Chemical drugs — ASPIRIN

1940s Antibiotics — PENICILLIN

1875 PUBLIC HEALTH ACT

1840s Anaesthetics
1860s ANTISEPSIS
1890s X-rays
1914 Blood transfusion

Increasingly complex surgery

1940s Plastic surgery
1960s Transplants
1980s Keyhole surgery

1750–1900

THE TWENTIETH CENTURY

1750   1900   AD2000

6.3 *Women in medicine – a case study in change and continuity*

The next four pages give you the chance to investigate changes and continuities in an important theme in medical history.

Women have always played a vital role in healing the sick. Mothers and wives have always looked after the sick in their families. Whenever extra help was needed, for centuries people turned to the local 'wise-woman'. In every town and village people trusted these wise-women because of their deep knowledge of herbs and other treatments.

However, women have not always been allowed to play a more official or professional role in medicine. When were women allowed to train to be doctors or midwives? Is this new or did it happen throughout history?

■ ACTIVITY

Copy this table. You are going to complete it using Sources 2–10 on pages 109–111. You can also look back through this book to get more information. The finished table will help you to answer question 3.

	Ancient Egypt	Ancient Greece	Ancient Rome	Middle Ages	1350– 1750	1750– 1900	1900– present
What kinds of medical work did women do?							
What were the attitudes to women working in medicine?							

1 Your first task is to complete the top row.
   a) Read Source 2 and fill in the Ancient Egypt column in the top row, saying what the source tells you about the medical work done by Egyptian women. Use Source 1 to help you.
   b) Now look at the other sources and complete the top row. There is more than one source for some of the columns.
2 Now complete the bottom row.
   a) Read Source 2 again. Fill in the Ancient Egypt column in the bottom row, saying what the source tells you about attitudes to women working in medicine.
   b) Now look at the other sources again and complete the bottom row. Again, there is more than one source for some of the columns.
3 a) What kinds of medical work did women do most often before 1750?
   b) Why do you think these were the most common kinds of work done by women?
   c) How did attitudes to women in medicine change from the 1600s?
   d) What was the result of this change in attitudes?

▼ **SOURCE 1** Medical work done by women outside the home at various times through history

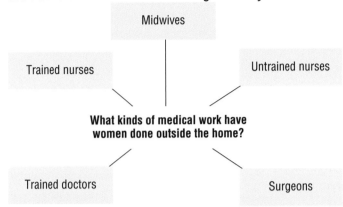

Midwives

Trained nurses

Untrained nurses

What kinds of medical work have women done outside the home?

Trained doctors

Surgeons

▼ **SOURCE 2** From a textbook on medicine in Ancient Egypt

A woman is listed among the healing priests. She was Peseshet who lived around 2500BC. She was the Lady Overseer of Lady Physicians. Only one other woman is listed among the 129 doctors known in Ancient Egypt.

▼ **SOURCE 3** Written by Hyginus, a Greek writer

The ancient Greeks had no midwives because they had decided that no women should learn the science of medicine. A girl called Hagnodice wanted to learn the science of medicine so she cut off her hair, put on men's clothing and went to Herophilus for training in medicine.

▶ **SOURCE 5** Midwives attending a birth in the Middle Ages. In some countries midwives had to have licences after qualifying through an apprenticeship. However, women could not become doctors because they were not allowed to go to university to study medicine. Women could also do simple surgery because surgery was learned through practice, not from books of theory

▼ **SOURCE 4** This is a drawing of a carving done nearly 2000 years ago in the second century AD. It shows a Roman midwife and her assistant delivering a baby. A Roman medical writer said that the best midwives were not just faultless at the task of delivering babies but also understood the theories of medicine and were well-trained

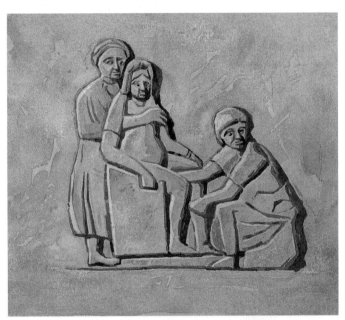

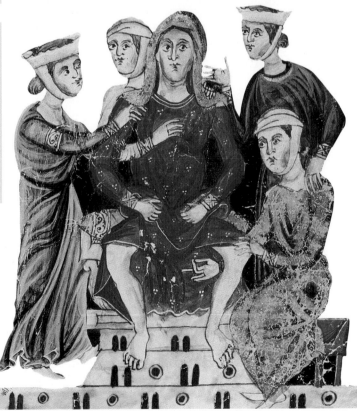

▼ **SOURCE 6** Records of the city of York, 1572. Male doctors had wished to stop Isabel Warwick treating the sick

[Isabel Warwick] has the skill in the science of surgery and has done good therein, it is therefore agreed that she, upon her good behaviour, shall use the same without obstruction by any of the surgeons of the city.

▼ **SOURCE 8** Florence Nightingale became famous as a nurse during the Crimean War in the 1850s. When she returned to Britain, she set up the first training school for nurses and improved conditions in hospitals. Because of her work, nursing became a respectable profession for young ladies and standards of nursing were greatly improved

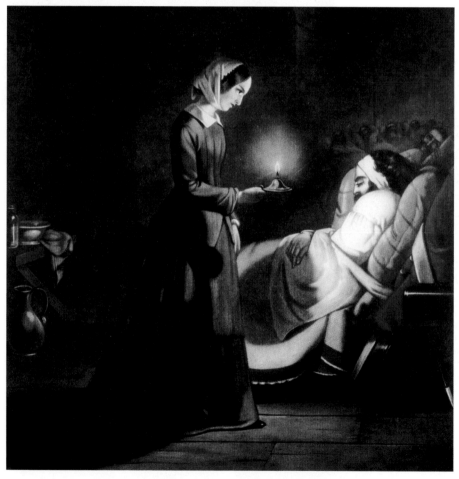

▼ **SOURCE 7** In 1620 Peter Chamberlan invented the obstetric forceps which helped to deliver babies. Over the next hundred years this invention lowered the status of women midwives. Some knowledge of anatomy was needed to use the forceps and only men were allowed to learn anatomy at university. Therefore, male doctors began to take over from midwives at some births. It also became fashionable for rich women to have male doctors instead of midwives

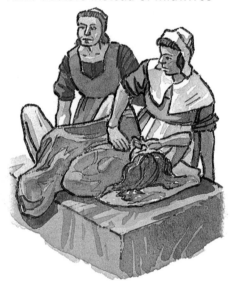

▶ **SOURCE 9** In 1865 Elizabeth Garrett became the first woman to qualify as a doctor in Britain. She had overcome many obstacles. Science was not taught to girls in schools. Her father thought that the idea of a woman doctor was disgusting. Male students protested about attending classes that were also attended by a woman. Universities would not give degrees to women. However, in 1876, a law was passed opening all medical qualifications to women

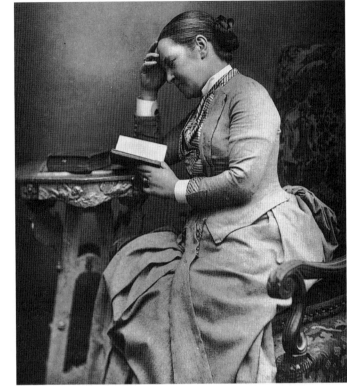

▼ **SOURCE 10** Nowadays many women train to be doctors. About 50 per cent of doctors qualifying in Britain every year are women

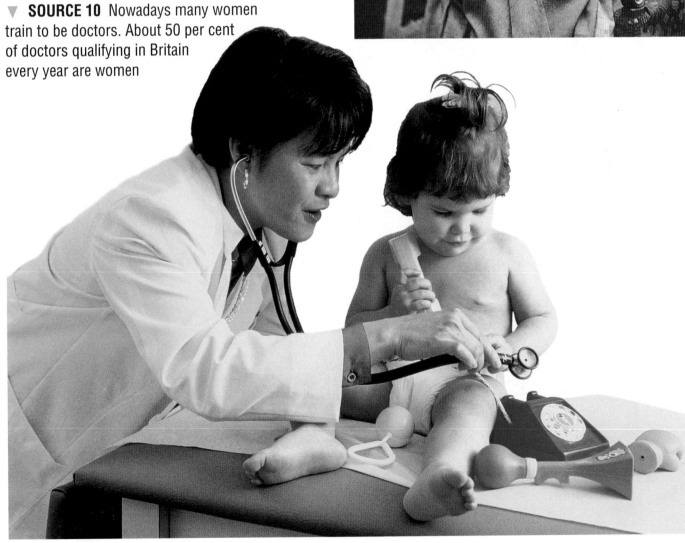

6.4 *Why? The factors that cause change and continuity*

■ ACTIVITY 1

Look at the factors shown in the picture below.

1 Attitudes and beliefs have had a major effect on the development of medicine. Which **two** people in the picture are examples of attitudes and beliefs?
2 Which other factor in this picture have you not met before? Can you think of an example in this book?
3 Look at the boxes opposite. Match each box to one of the factors in the picture below.

4 Using boxes 1–6 and the rest of the book, list two ways in which each factor affected the history of medicine.
5 For each factor, explain whether it led to change or continuity or both in the history of medicine.
6 Which factors do you think have been the most important in the history of medicine for:
   a) causing change
   b) maintaining continuity?

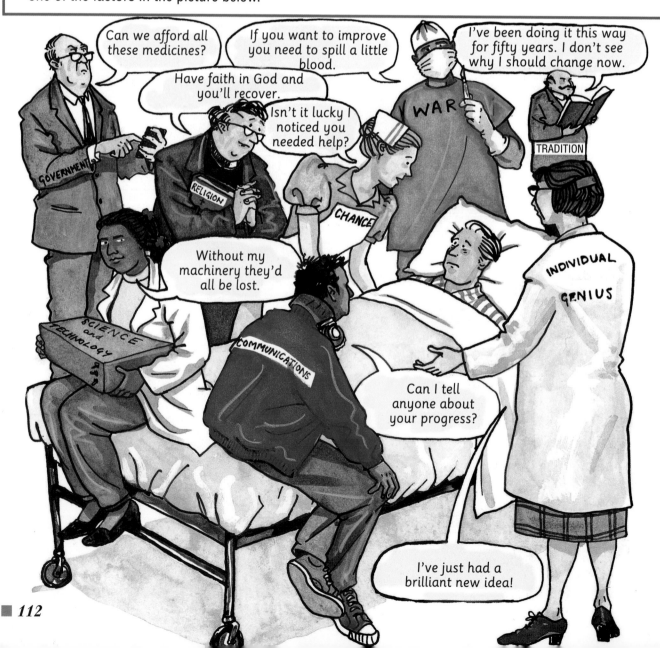

1
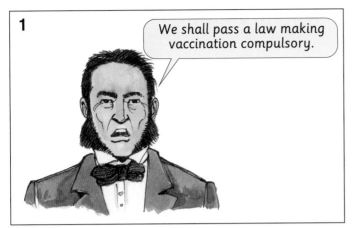
We shall pass a law making vaccination compulsory.

2
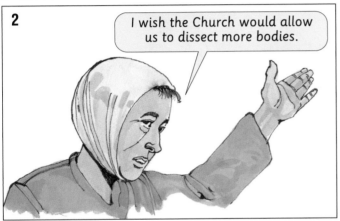
I wish the Church would allow us to dissect more bodies.

3
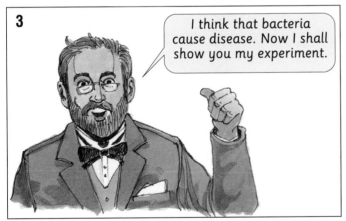
I think that bacteria cause disease. Now I shall show you my experiment.

4
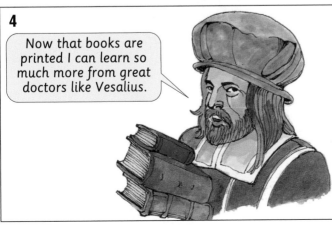
Now that books are printed I can learn so much more from great doctors like Vesalius.

5
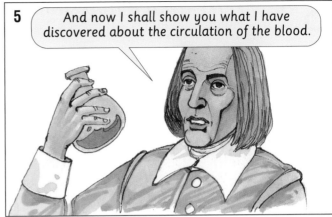
And now I shall show you what I have discovered about the circulation of the blood.

6
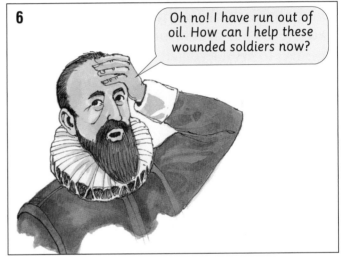
Oh no! I have run out of oil. How can I help these wounded soldiers now?

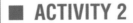

■ ACTIVITY 2

7 Individuals have made important contributions to the development of medicine. Choose one of the following individuals:

- Andreas Vesalius
- Joseph Lister
- James Simpson
- Alexander Fleming.

For the individual you have chosen:
a) Briefly explain the contribution he made to the development of medicine.
b) Were his ideas welcomed by people at the time? Explain your answer.
c) Was individual brilliance the only reason why he was able to make an important contribution to the development of medicine? Explain your answer.

6.5 *Why do we live so much longer nowadays?*

The last pages – and the answers to our big question!

For thousands of years most people died before they were 40. In the 1800s people began to live a little longer and by 1900 the average life expectancy had reached 50. By 2001 this had increased much more rapidly, to well over 70. On these pages you can see how the doors to a longer life have been opened.

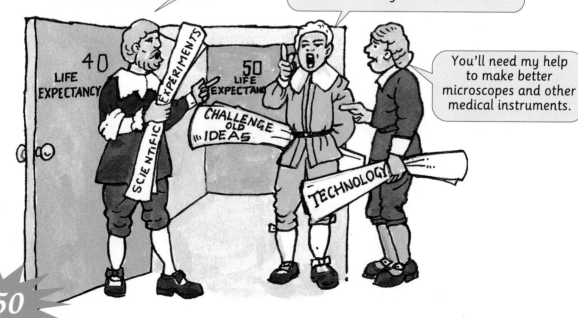

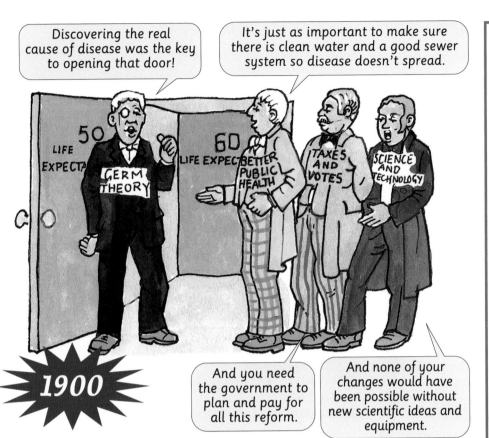

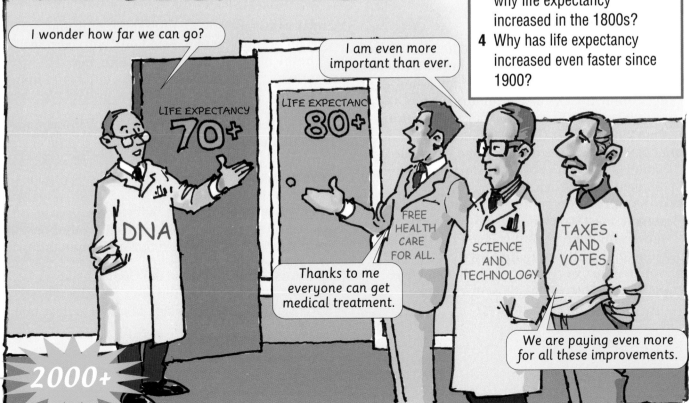

■ ACTIVITY

Use the questions below to help you to write a short essay answering the question 'Why do we live so much longer nowadays?'

Your essay will contain four paragraphs. Each paragraph is to be based on one of the four illustrations on these two pages. Begin each paragraph with the answer to one of the questions below. Then add in more detail using the illustrations to help you.

1 Why were there very few new ideas about medicine in the Middle Ages around 1350?
2 Which vital step forward in medicine had happened by 1750?
3 What were the main reasons why life expectancy increased in the 1800s?
4 Why has life expectancy increased even faster since 1900?

Glossary

ABSCESS a collection of pus caused by an infection

AD *Anno Domini*, a Latin term meaning 'In the year of our Lord'. It is used in the Christian calendar to describe dates after the birth of Jesus

AMPUTATE to cut off a damaged arm, leg, hand or foot

ANAESTHETIC a drug given to patients to put them into a deep sleep so that they feel no pain during an operation

ANATOMY the parts that make up the body; also the study of how the body is made up

ANTIBIOTIC a drug used to kill the bacteria that cause infections; the first to be artificially manufactured was penicillin

ANTIBODIES proteins produced in the blood to fight harmful organisms

ANTISEPSIS the destruction of unwanted organisms

ANTISEPTICS chemicals used to kill bacteria and prevent infection

AQUEDUCT a channel used to carry clean water to towns; they were an important part of Roman public health schemes

ASEPTIC a germ-free state

BACTERIA germs that cause infection and disease

BC 'Before Christ', used in the Christian calendar to describe dates before the birth of Jesus; dates are counted backwards from the birth of Jesus so 4000BC is 2000 years further back in time than 2000BC

BLEEDING releasing blood from a cut made in a patient's body, in order to restore the balance of the body's humours

BLOOD GROUP the particular type of blood that a person has; blood transfusions are only successful if the patient is given the type of blood that matches his/her own

BLOOD TRANSFUSION giving fresh blood to a patient to replace blood lost during an operation or through injury

CARBOLIC SPRAY carbolic acid, used as a disinfectant and antiseptic

CAUTERISE to burn a wound in order to prevent infection and excess bleeding

CELL the smallest part of an organism that is able to function on its own

CESSPOOL a place where sewage collects

CHARM an object believed to have magical powers to cure or prevent sickness

CHLOROFORM an early type of anaesthetic

CHOLERA a disease carried in water contaminated by sewage. It causes violent sickness and diarrhoea and usually leads to the victim's death

CULTURE micro-organisms (tiny living things) grown in a laboratory for use in experiments

DELIRIOUS excited and confused, as a result of a high fever

DIAGNOSIS the doctor's opinion about what is wrong with a patient (plural DIAGNOSES)

DIAPHRAGM the large sheet of muscle separating the chest from the abdomen

DISSECT to cut open a body and examine the insides

EMBALMING removing internal organs and treating the skin of a dead body with certain chemicals to prevent it from decaying

EPIDEMIC a disease that spreads quickly to many people

GENE a section of DNA that contains information about a particular characteristic, e.g. hair or eye colour

GENETIC ENGINEERING changing the way genes work in the body

GERM a micro-organism that causes disease

GLADIATORS people who fought each other or wild animals as entertainment during Roman times

HUMOURS four fluids that the Greeks believed were important in keeping the body healthy. These were blood, phlegm, black bile and yellow bile

IMMUNISE   to protect against disease, often by vaccination

IMMUNITY   the ability of an organism to resist disease

INOCULATE   to inject a person with a tiny amount of bacteria that cause a particular disease. The body then develops immunity to the bacteria and so the person will not become too ill if they catch the disease

LIFE EXPECTANCY   the length of time that a person can expect to live

LIGATURE   a thread used to tie off blood vessels to prevent excess bleeding

MALARIA   a disease carried by mosquitoes, especially common in warm, marshy areas

MEDIEVAL   from the Middle Ages (AD1000–1500)

MIDWIFE   someone who is skilled in dealing with pregnancy and childbirth

MONASTERY   a building in which monks live, work and pray

NATIONAL HEALTH SERVICE (NHS)   the system in which the government uses money from taxes to pay for health care, so that individual patients do not have to pay when they need to see a doctor or have an operation, etc.

OBSERVE   to watch carefully

PAPYRUS   an early type of paper made from reeds, used by the Egyptians

PATENT MEDICINES   herbal remedies that were sold in shops and were protected by a patent (registered) so no one else could copy them. They were usually worthless.

PHARAOH   an Egyptian king

PHYSICIAN   a doctor

PILLORY   a wooden framework with holes for the head and hands, used as punishment. Other people could shout at the person imprisoned and throw things at them.

PLAGUE   a serious disease passed to humans by fleas carried on rats; the word was also used in early times to mean any serious disease

PLASTIC SURGERY   the repair of missing, unformed or injured tissue or body parts

PNEUMONIA   inflammation of the lungs caused by an infection

PUBLIC HEALTH   the health of the general population. It also means measures taken to improve the health of the population, such as supplying clean drinking water

PURGE   to get rid of everything that has been eaten; a medicine to do this

RATIONING   the system introduced during the Second World War to make sure that food was shared out fairly

REMEDY   something that cures sickness

REVOLUTION   a big change in the way people live and work, or in the way they are governed

SHRAPNEL   a bomb containing material that explodes before impact

SKIN GRAFT   a piece of skin removed from one part of the body to repair an injury or burn

SLUMS   very poor housing with few or no services such as running water and toilets

SMALLPOX   a serious disease, which was a common killer until a vaccine was discovered in the late eighteenth century

SURGEON   a doctor who performs operations

SURGERY   treating a patient by performing an operation on them

VACCINE   something that is injected (by VACCINATION) into the body to make the body produce antibodies and so protect it against disease

VIRUS   a particle living in the cells of animals that causes disease

X-RAYS   pictures of the inside of the body

Index